To Improve Health and Health Care

Volume XIII

Stephen L. Isaacs and
David C. Colby, Editors
Foreword by Risa Lavizzo-Mourey

—ᴡᴡ—To Improve Health and Health Care

Volume XIII

The Robert Wood Johnson
Foundation Anthology

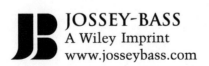
JOSSEY-BASS
A Wiley Imprint
www.josseybass.com

Published by Jossey-Bass
A Wiley Imprint
989 Market Street, San Francisco, CA 94103-1741—www.josseybass.com

Jossey-Bass books and products are available through most bookstores. To contact Jossey-Bass directly call our Customer Care Department within the U.S. at 800-956-7739, outside the U.S. at 317-572-3986, or fax 317-572-4002.

Jossey-Bass also publishes its books in a variety of electronic formats. Some content that appears in print may not be available in electronic books.

ISSN: 1547-3570
ISBN 10: 0-4704-9663-0
ISBN 13: 978-04704-9663-3

Printed in the United States of America
FIRST EDITION
PB Printing 10 9 8 7 6 5 4 3 2 1

—ᴡ—Contents

We dedicate this volume of the Anthology *to the memory of two giants in the field who passed away in 2009*

Terrance Keenan (1924–2009)

Compassionate leader, visionary grant maker, mentor to many, and great friend

Frank Karel (1935–2009)

Preeminent thinker, who revolutionized philanthropic communications; gifted intellect and story teller; warm and gracious friend

Both men touched many lives. They shall be missed.

—ᴠᴠ—Foreword

Risa Lavizzo-Mourey

One of the challenges for any organization striving to be great is to look—systematically and objectively—into activities that it has undertaken, acknowledge those that did not meet expectations, and draw lessons from them for the future. This does not come easily to any organization; it is especially difficult for foundations. When I first became the president and chief executive officer of the Robert Wood Johnson Foundation, my predecessor, Steven Schroeder, reminded me that there are no external forces compelling foundations to examine their work and assess what worked and what didn't; the motivation has to be internal, to come from a desire to achieve excellence.

This volume of the *Anthology* features four chapters that take a hard look at programs that did not work out as planned. Three of the chapters examine why the programs did not meet our expectations and draw lessons for future Foundation programming. The fourth chapter is a commentary by Bob Hughes, a Foundation vice president and its chief learning officer. I draw four general lessons of my own from this section of the *Anthology*.

First, when we look back at programs that did not meet expectations, we must be reflective and respectful. We must recognize that no one ever sets out to have something fail and that everyone who works on a program comes at it with a sense of commitment to bringing about social change. We must honor and respect that commitment.

Second, we must be balanced in our approach, and understand gradations and nuance. I do not think that we could ever come up with a perfect project, nor find one that was a complete and utter failure. Most projects fall between these two extremes.

Third, the impact of programs may change over time. Initial success may fade with time or without intensive cultivation by Foundation staff. Failing programs, as Tony Proscio points out, may become successful after midcourse corrections. Some good ideas that are not widely adopted or are blocked by powerful forces become the great innovations of the next generation. Foundations such as ours have the unique privilege of being able to take the longer view.

Fourth, we must place programs in the context of the strategic goals and objectives set out in our impact framework. In examining programs that disappointed, we should consider them in the context of what we can learn about the effectiveness of our overall strategy. For that is what we are trying to do—to understand programs, both individually and collectively, and their level of success and place them in the context of what we can do to achieve social change in health and health care.

As a foundation, we are dedicated to learning from our past activities. Our Guiding Principles, which state, "We must be objective, rigorous, and transparent in assessing grantees' progress and the results of their work" and "We must commit ourselves to lifelong learning and continual improvement," reinforce an internal culture of improvement. We honor that commitment through our Grant Results Reports, our outside evaluations of national programs, our annual scorecard, and the publication of the *Anthology* series. The chapters on programs that did not work out as planned illustrate our commitment to learning and improvement. I hope that they will provide guidance not only to the Robert Wood Johnson Foundation but to the field of philanthropy as well.

—〰—EDITORS' INTRODUCTION

David C. Colby and Stephen L. Isaacs

Last year, we decided to devote several chapters of the *Anthology* to a single theme—the Robert Wood Johnson Foundation's efforts to advance health reform. This year's *Anthology* addresses a different theme, focusing on learning from programs that did not work out as planned. As Risa Lavizzo-Mourey observes in her foreword, at a time when foundations are becoming more aware of the need to be publicly accountable, it is important to report on programs that haven't worked, as well as those that have.

Thus, the first section is devoted to learning from programs that did not meet expectations. Chapter 1, by the editors of the *Anthology*, is an overview of the topic. It examines a number of different programs that, for a variety of reasons, did not achieve their objectives. It is followed by a chapter written by Tony Proscio that examines several programs that underwent major adjustments even as they were underway. The third chapter, by Michael Brown, looks at a single program that went awry. The section concludes, in chapter 4, with a commentary by Robert Hughes, a vice president of the Robert Wood Johnson Foundation and its chief learning officer, that pulls together lessons from the three preceding chapters.

The next section, aimed at giving readers a greater understanding of the Robert Wood Johnson Foundation and how it operates, contains a single chapter. In chapter 5, David Morse and Fred Mann, the vice president and assistant vice president, respectively, of communications at the Foundation, trace the evolution of the Foundation's communications strategy from one of working through grantees to one of working collaboratively with grantees. It provides an inside perspective on how the Foundation adapted its communications approach to keep up with changing times and new Foundation priorities.

The next three chapters explore Foundation-funded initiatives to improve addiction prevention and treatment. In chapter 6, James Bornemeier provides an overview of the Foundation's efforts to reduce addiction to drugs. In chapter 7, Sara Solovitch examines Reclaiming Futures, a program aimed at changing the way prevention and treatment services are offered to young people in the juvenile justice system addicted to alcohol or drugs. The eighth chapter, by Lee Green, looks at the College Alcohol Study, which focused national attention on binge drinking by college students.

The final section contains two chapters examining Foundation-funded initiatives to improve health and health care. In chapter 9, Irene Wielawski describes the Foundation's efforts through the Hablamos Juntos program to reduce language barriers faced by Spanish-speaking patients. In the last chapter, Digby Diehl describes the MicheLee Puppets troupe and its efforts to educate Florida schoolchildren about how to eat better and live healthier lives.

Readers of the *Anthology* may be interested in knowing that the editors, too, are keeping up with the times. An enhanced version of the *Anthology* series now appears on the Robert Wood Johnson Foundation Web site, www.rwjf.org, and individual chapters can be easily downloaded, reprinted, and distributed. There is also an interactive link through which readers can communicate with the editors or comment on individual chapters in this volume and earlier ones.

—᭡—Acknowledgments

It takes a substantial community more than a year to write, edit, and produce the Robert Wood Johnson Foundation *Anthology*. We wish to acknowledge the contribution of the members of that community.

The process begins in the spring with the editors' selection of topics for the next *Anthology*. Topics are frequently based on suggestions made by the Foundation's staff members, either informally via hall conversations or e-mails or more formally in a meeting of the program staff. The editors commission authors for each of the chapters and ask Foundation staff members to gather materials that will get the authors started. Rose Littman, Sarah Pickell, and Diane Martinez were extremely diligent in digging out material, as were members of the Foundation's Information Center: Hinda Greenberg, Mary Beth Kren, and Barbara Sergeant. When draft chapters arrive months later, the editors often ask Foundation staff members or knowledgeable outsiders to review them. We thank Nancy Barrand, Pam Dickson, Lori Grubstein, Jim Ingram, Michelle Larkin, Connie Pechura, Kristin Schubert, and Steve Schroeder for their thoughtful comments on specific chapters.

In February, the outside review committee gathers in Princeton to review the draft chapters. That committee—comprised of Susan Dentzer, Bill Morrill, Patti Patrizi, and Jon Showstack—performs an invaluable function, and every chapter in the book is improved thanks to the efforts its members. Pat Crow serves as executive editor of the *Anthology* series, and Molly McKaughan checks the manuscript for accuracy concerning Foundation strategy and implementation. Lauren MacIntyre converts Pat Crow's handwritten edits into a Word format. Carolyn Shea carefully fact-checks every chapter, giving us confidence that facts and quotations are accurate. Within the Foundation, members of the Office of Program Management—Patti Higgins, Lydia Ryba, Kathleen McGeady, and Richard Toth—give us similar confidence regarding Foundation-related program and financial information.

Prior to our submitting it to Jossey-Bass, Risa Lavizzo-Mourey and David Morse review the entire manuscript. They also provide wise guidance to the editors throughout the process, for which we are grateful. Fred Mann and Adam Coyne serve as trusted counselors with whom we discuss ideas and issues as the book is being developed.

A number of people contribute to the *Anthology*'s development from beginning to end. At Health Policy Associates, Elizabeth Dawson manages the entire research and editorial process and, in addition, handles administrative matters, and Jay Franz does the bookkeeping associated with the *Anthology*. At the Robert Wood Johnson Foundation, Mimi Turi, Mary Castria, Carol Owle, Carolyn Scholer, and Chris Sowa manage contractual and financial matters, and Deb Malloy, Sherry DeMarchi, Chris Clayton, and Tina Hines keep arrangements between the San Francisco-based editor and the Foundation staff flowing smoothly.

At the production and marketing level, we acknowledge the efforts of Andy Pasternack, Kelsey McGee, and Seth Schwartz at Jossey-Bass. At the Robert Wood Johnson Foundation, Hope Woodhead oversees production matters, and she and Barbara Sherwood handle mailing and distribution. Larry Blumenthal and Penny Bolla make the pages of the Foundation's Web site where *Anthology* chapters are posted far more user-friendly and easy to navigate.

To the entire community of people who make the *Anthology* series possible, we express our profound gratitude.

DCC and SLI

To Improve Health and Health Care

Volume XIII

Section One

Learning from Programs that Did Not Work Out as Planned

Editors' Introduction to Section One

Learning from Programs that Did Not Work Out as Planned

The first four chapters of this year's *Anthology* are devoted to programs that did not work out as planned and what can be learned from them. The first chapter, written by the editors of the *Anthology,* examines eight programs that disappointed because they were either conceptually flawed, ran up against strong social or political headwinds, or were poorly executed. While these are not the only Foundation-funded programs that failed to meet expectations, they offer a representative sample and allow us to extract lessons that might prove useful in future programming by the Robert Wood Johnson Foundation and other foundations.

The second chapter, written by Tony Proscio, a freelance writer and consultant to foundations and nonprofit organizations, looks at programs that were going off track and underwent mid-course corrections. Unlike the programs discussed in the first chapter, the programs that Proscio examines were assessed early and adjustments to them were made. This chapter is unusual in that the author and the editors decided to disguise the grantees in the last of the three case studies. The difficult decision to conceal the names of the programs was made because some of the participants are still working in the field, and we felt that naming them might have damaged their reputations without conferring any strong counterbalancing benefit. While transparency is certainly a desirable goal, in practice, as this chapter illustrates, it is not always easy to achieve. There is a difference between opening oneself to public scrutiny and airing sensitive matters that could be harmful, and that difference must be recognized and respected.

The third chapter, by Michael H. Brown, a freelance writer and former reporter for the *Louisville Courier-Journal,* offers an in-depth examination of a single program, the National Health Care Purchasing Institute. A great deal went wrong in the planning, oversight, and execution of the initiative. Ultimately, the Foundation terminated its support ahead of schedule and transferred the remaining funds from one grantee to another. As Brown recounts it, this is a story of confusion of purpose, disagreement both internally and among the various participants, poor communications, and precipitous program termination. All told, not a particularly pretty tale, and the editors (and others at the Robert Wood Johnson Foundation) debated whether to make it public. In the final analysis, the value of the piece to the field persuaded us to publish the chapter.

The fourth chapter, a commentary by Robert G. Hughes, a Foundation vice president and its chief learning officer, pulls together themes from the three preceding chapters. Unlike the editors and the authors, Hughes does not shy away from using the word "failure." He makes the case that, difficult as it may be, recognizing failure and calling it by its proper name is imperative if foundations are to learn from their program experiences. In Hughes' own words, "Critical and honest examinations of their work will help foundations become more realistic about impact and more effective at fulfilling their contributions to society."

CHAPTER 1

Good Ideas at the Time: Learning from Programs that Did Not Work Out as Expected

Stephen L. Isaacs and David C. Colby

Unwelcome as the news might sometimes be, there is as much to learn from foundation programs that fail to meet expectations as there is from programs that have met or exceeded them—perhaps more. The truth is that not every program can succeed as planned. "There have to be programs that don't work out," said Tracy Orleans, distinguished fellow and senior scientist at the Robert Wood Johnson Foundation. "If there aren't, we are not doing our job—we are not taking enough risk." Thus, it is not surprising that some Foundation-funded programs that seemed like good ideas at the time have not turned out to be so in practice.

The important thing is to learn from those programs that have not met expectations. A first step is trying to understand why programs did not work out as planned. Our review of

Foundation-funded programs that did not meet expectations*
identified three primary reasons that they did not succeed:

The first is flawed strategy or design. Goals may be unrealistic
or unreachable. Objectives may be unclear, or even conflicting.
Various participants may have different ideas about what the goals
are. Or the goal may be sound but the strategies to reach them
problematic or unworkable.

The second is a difficult environmental context. Though the
goals may be worthy, society is simply not ready for them or they
may not be politically feasible. Or conditions at the planning stage
are overtaken by economic, political, or social events, rendering
even a well-conceived program ineffective in practice.

The third is faulty execution. There are myriad reasons that
programs are not implemented effectively—lack of management
ability, poor interpersonal relations skills, flawed leadership, bad
judgment, and intra-organizational controversy, to name just
a few.

In practice, it isn't easy to single out design flaws, execution
flaws, or societal challenges as *the* factors that cause a program
to disappoint; more than one of these are often present. Nor
is it always possible to know when a program has not worked
out: Muddy goals or strategies make it difficult to determine
effectiveness. Moreover, program outcomes are rarely 100 percent
positive or 100 percent negative. "It is not just a matter of
success versus failure," said Nancy Barrand, the special adviser for
program development at the Robert Wood Johnson Foundation.
"You've got to account for the shades of gray."

As important as understanding why programs have not lived
up to expectations is drawing lessons from them. This involves
learning how to identify problems early and, where possible,

---

* These are programs that outside evaluators or Foundation staff members have
found did not meet expectations, not just those that in the authors' opinion
failed to reach their potential.

addressing them in a timely manner, as well as using the lessons from disappointing efforts in the design of new programs.

—᷈᷈— Programs that Did Not Meet Expectations Primarily Because of Strategic or Design Flaws

Strategic grant making of the sort that the Robert Wood Johnson Foundation and other large national foundations practice usually begins with setting goals and developing strategies to reach them. "I think the problems start with a lack of clarity about what you're trying to accomplish," Paul Brest, the president of The William and Flora Hewlett Foundation, said in a recent interview. "If you're not clear about what the goals are, it's really hard to know if you've succeeded. Beyond that, you need to have a plan to get there—a theory of change or logic model that links your philanthropic interventions to the goals you want to achieve. But it has to be realistic."

Three Robert Wood Johnson Foundation-funded programs that did not meet expectations primarily because of flawed strategy or design are Community Programs for Affordable Health Care, Best Friends, and the Health Professions Partnership Initiative.

Community Programs for Affordable Health Care

In the early 1980s, many health policy experts looked to Rochester, New York, as a model for curbing spiraling health costs. In Rochester, employers, hospitals, and insurers had formed a voluntary coalition to cut health care costs by enrolling people in managed care. Staff members at the Robert Wood Johnson Foundation thought it worthwhile to try a similar voluntary, community-wide approach in other cities. So when the American Hospital Association and The Blue Cross Blue Shield Foundation proposed an idea to develop socially responsible cost containment programs in other American cities, the Foundation responded positively with Community Programs for Affordable

Health Care (CPAHC), a $16.2 million initiative that began, in 1983, to test cost-containment strategies in eleven locations. The program embodied, as one commentator noted, "an idealistic, sunny notion ... that community representatives holding very different vested interests would voluntarily put aside their own needs and aspirations to find a solution to a problem for the greater good."[1]

Almost as soon as it began, the program began to unravel. Foundation staff members became wary that the high-powered national advisory committee was taking the program in directions that the Foundation had not anticipated and did not approve of. "The national advisory committee thought that the Foundation had given it a blank check and that they were supposed to figure out how to spend it," said Alan Cohen, a former Foundation vice president who had arrived after the program was under way but in time to oversee the evaluation. "We were sitting and watching and couldn't believe what was happening." The national program office also managed the program in ways that troubled the Foundation's staff. "One potential grantee was so upset at the management style of the first national program director that it turned down the award," Cohen recalled. Perhaps because the community partners were often joined in shotgun marriages, the programs they developed, in the judgment of Foundation officials, were pegged to the least common acceptable denominator and totally uninspired. So concerned was the Foundation's board that in 1986 it rescinded $3 million that had been authorized but not yet expended for the program.

The outside evaluators, Lawrence Brown, a Columbia University political scientist, and Catherine McLaughlin, a University of Michigan economist, skewered Community Programs for Affordable Health Care in an article in *Health Affairs*. "The basic reason why the CPAHC mission did not succeed is that it was always 'mission impossible,'" they wrote. "The key policy lesson of CPAHC, and its major contribution to the national policy debate, is to demonstrate ... the bankruptcy of [the notions] that communities can and should be awarded a leadership role in containing health care costs, that progress is inevitable if only the leaders of powerful local health care institutions come to the bargaining table...and that government and the market must be held at bay."[2] Senior Foundation staff members agreed that a flawed strategy had sunk the program. "The program's central flaw, perhaps," wrote Alan Cohen, Joel Cantor, and Steven Schroeder, "was its misguided assumption that cost containment could be achieved through intervention at the community or local level, when the true levers of power and control existed (and still exist) at the national level and state levels."[3]

John Dunlop, the chairman of the national advisory committee, and George Stiles, executive director of the Council on Health Costs, which was the program's grantee in Charlotte, North Carolina, disagreed. "CPAHC's objectives were more modest and focused than the Brown and McLaughlin caricature," they wrote. "It is ludicrous to believe...that the modest CPAHC resources could demonstrate major community-wide savings (especially in larger cities such as New York and Detroit) in four years or less."[4]

Donald Cohodes, a high-ranking Blue Cross Blue Shield Association official who directed CPAHC for fourteen months in 1985 and 1986, added his two cents' worth, calling the program a "design failure"[5]—one whose objectives were unrealistic and should not have been tried in the first place. This may be unduly harsh. At the time the program was being developed, health care costs were spinning out of control, Rochester seemed to have found a way of containing them, and nothing else seemed to be working. Why not try something new, even something that might be a long shot? The design flaw was both in trying to address a national problem at the local level and in assuming that an experiment in one city, Rochester, which had a unique environment (a few dominant corporations, a single major health insurer, and a limited number of hospitals), could be replicated in American cities with wholly different characteristics. Since the program appeared to have been badly mismanaged, even though flaws in the design may be the primary reason it did not succeed, poor execution contributed as well.

Probably the main lesson is that foundations entering the rough-and-tumble world of local politics should do so with their eyes wide open and be aware that local politics can be venal. In the words of Brown and McLaughlin, foundation-funded programs aimed at containing costs "always threaten the earnings, mission, or autonomy (or all three) of major health care interests."[6] More broadly, CPAHC represents something of a loss of innocence about the potential of local coalitions to be the engines of policy change and of the capacity of foundations to contain the cost of medical care.

Best Friends

Even from the start, the Best Friends program was a stretch. A "character-building" program for sixth- through eighth-grade girls from low-income neighborhoods,[7] Best Friends promotes an abstinence-only approach to sex and also to drugs and alcohol. In the words of Elayne Bennett, a Georgetown University educator, co-founder of the program, and wife of former Education Secretary William Bennett, Best Friends "promotes self-respect through the practice of self-control and provides participants [with] the skills, guidance, and support to choose abstinence from sex until marriage and reject illegal drug and alcohol use."[8]

A controversial, unproven approach, abstinence only has been criticized as unworkable and out of touch with reality—even damaging, since it denies potentially sexually active girls access to information on ways other than abstaining to avoid becoming pregnant. Not that anybody is against abstinence before marriage. But there is, as Sarah Brown, executive director of the National Campaign to Prevent Teen Pregnancy, a Foundation grantee between 1997 and 2008, noted, "a profound difference between abstinence as a *message* and abstinence-only *interventions*."[9]

Between 1990 and 2003, the Robert Wood Johnson Foundation awarded five grants totaling $2.2 million to enable the Best Friends Foundation to carry out Best Friends programs in schools across the country. The programs followed the same general format in all the schools: an eight-session curriculum given throughout the school year; mentoring by a faculty member; participation in a weekly fitness or dance class; fulfillment of a community service requirement; various cultural enrichment activities; and scholarships to help program participants attend college or graduate school. By the end of the grant period in 2003, school systems were operating Best Friends programs in twenty-three cities in fourteen states, the District of Columbia, and the US Virgin Islands, with nearly 5,000 girls participating.[10]

In 1996, Congress passed the Personal Responsibility and Work Opportunity Reconciliation Act (the law reforming welfare), which significantly increased funding for programs that teach "abstinence from sexual activity outside of marriage as the expected standard for school age children." The following year, Congress authorized an evaluation of these abstinence-education programs. The evaluation was to be carried out by Mathematica Policy Research, a New Jersey-based research and evaluation firm. Wanting to add some Best Friends sites to the federal evaluation, the Robert Wood Johnson Foundation, in November 1999, awarded a $750,000 six-year grant to Mathematica to evaluate Best Friends.

Shortly thereafter, the evaluation plan started to come apart. The Best Friends Foundation, on the one side, and the Robert Wood Johnson Foundation and Mathematica, on the other, were unable to agree upon a plan to evaluate the program. A series of meetings of the leaders of the three organizations revealed disagreement on such fundamental issues as the evaluation methodology and the outcomes that should be measured. James Knickman, who was the Robert Wood Johnson Foundation vice president for research and evaluation at the time, recalled, "We wanted to take a random survey of students who had enrolled in the program;

Best Friends said no. Best Friends wanted to discard any girl from the survey who had had sex; we felt this was unworkable." A stalemate ensued; the Best Friends Foundation refused to participate in the Foundation-funded evaluation. In January 2000, the Robert Wood Johnson Foundation cancelled the evaluation, and shortly thereafter Mathematica returned its initial payment for the study. The Foundation continued funding the Best Friends program through 2003, the end of the grant period.

Seven years after the Best Friends' evaluation was terminated, Mathematica published its evaluation of four abstinence-only programs funded by the federal government. The results showed the abstinence-only approach to be ineffective.[11]

In hindsight, it would not be unreasonable to question the decision to fund Best Friends, since the Foundation does not usually support programs employing approaches that have no evidence whatsoever of being effective. At the time the program was developed, however, there was great concern about the high rate of adolescent pregnancy and a desire to try a variety of approaches, including abstinence-only ones, to reduce it. Since Best Friends appeared to be the most promising of the abstinence-only programs and appealed to political conservatives, it was considered the sort of long shot worth placing a small bet on.

A number of lessons emerge from the Best Friends' experience. One is the importance of investigating whether a strategy has *some* chance of working; that is, of assessing upfront the potential of the strategy to succeed. Equally important is the need to synchronize evaluation and program development at an early stage, where possible. Seven years elapsed before the Foundation decided to evaluate Best Friends. If the Best Friends program had been viewed as a test of an experimental approach to prevent teenage pregnancy—one that would be carefully evaluated—then there could have been an agreed-upon evaluation plan at the outset. Or it would have been clear that agreement on an evaluation could not be reached, and the decision whether to fund the program would have been considered in that light.

The Health Professions Partnership Initiative

Having funded programs throughout the 1970s and 1980s to prepare minority college students to be stronger candidates for medical school, the Foundation reached further down the pipeline in the 1990s to attract and prepare minority elementary and high school students for careers as physicians and other health professionals. In 1991, The Association of American Medical Colleges (AAMC) had initiated Project 3000 by 2000 with the goal of roughly doubling the number of underrepresented minorities (defined as blacks, Mexican Americans, mainland Puerto Ricans, and Native Americans) enrolled in medical schools. In 1994, the Foundation developed the Health Professions Partnership Initiative to support the AAMC in its Project 3000 by 2000. The idea behind the Health Professions Partnership Initiative was to increase the number of students from underrepresented minorities entering careers in both medicine and other health professions by creating a pre-medical pipeline below the college level. The program was designed to help medical and other health professions' schools build partnerships with secondary schools, colleges, and communities that would improve the quality of math and science teaching and increase, through enrichment activities, student interest in health careers.

The means adopted were ones that the Foundation had traditionally employed. It funded a number of different sites to come up with projects to attract and assist minority students, and it relied on local coalitions to carry out the projects. Initially, the coalitions were to revolve around medical schools, which were the grantees, and colleges, local schools, and school districts. Shortly after the initial ten grants were awarded, in 1996, the W.K. Kellogg Foundation agreed to co-fund the program. Since the Kellogg Foundation gave high priority to community-based initiatives, the two foundations stipulated that community organizations would be part of any coalitions formed for a second round of funding, in 1998. At the time of the third round of funding, schools of public health were added to the partnership mix.

All told, a total of twenty-six partnership programs were funded between 1996 and 2005, including five targeted to schools of public health. The lead agency was either a medical or other health professions school; partners were the public schools, community agencies, and in some cases the larger university. Each site received $70,000 per year for five years, and all the partners were expected to contribute resources toward the program.

The program, which ended in 2005, was evaluated by a team from the University of Washington School of Medicine. The evaluation team and informed observers from the AAMC found that, on the whole, the program did not meet expectations. The authors of the evaluation wrote that they were "unable to identify outcomes in terms of numbers of children influenced by programs or instances in which lasting changes in health professions schools had occurred."[12]

Some of the reasons that the program did not work out as expected had to do with its design, especially the strategies adopted to increase the number of minority high school students who would become doctors or other health professionals.

According to Jan Carline, the evaluator, and Davis Patterson, a research assistant associated with the evaluation, the foundations had unrealistic expectations about what small local interventions could accomplish in large complex public education systems working with seriously disadvantaged children. "The most effective methods for increasing the number of students academically capable of entering health careers appear to be based in general and systemic reform of education from the earliest levels of primary school through high school," they wrote. "A single intervention in one grade or school level or a series of unconnected interventions will not result in a sustainable increase in academic performance."[13]

Nor did the Robert Wood Johnson Foundation and the Kellogg Foundation understand public education very well. "Many of the failed programs did not take into account the difficult issues facing public schools today," Ella Cleveland, the program's deputy director at the AAMC, wrote in a 2006 supplement of *Academic Medicine* devoted to the Health Professions Partnership Initiative.[14]

The foundations also had unrealistic expectations about the ease of forming community partnerships and their effectiveness. In practice, forming effective coalitions turned out to be very difficult.[15]

The goals of the two foundations underwriting the program were never wholly compatible. The Robert Wood Johnson Foundation's goal sought to support coalitions built around academic health centers. The Kellogg Foundation emphasized the importance of community organizations.

Other reasons for the initiative's lack of success had to do with the changing perceptions of race and education. "During the project, institutions of higher learning were buffeted by a series of legal, legislative, and ballot-based setbacks to affirmative action," Charles Terrell, who directed the program at the AAMC between 2002 and 2005, wrote. "The tragic impact of these imposed barriers was that *Project 3000 by 2000* did not meet its goal."[16] Moreover, the initiative was underfunded. "One of the most important factors," Jane Lowe, who currently directs the Foundation's vulnerable populations team, said, "was the lack of funds to get the job done. Seventy-thousand dollars a year barely paid for a staff person." Finally, the execution of the program did not proceed smoothly. At the national program office, the key person at the AAMC died early in the program, and it took a long time to replace him. At project sites, leadership within some of the communities proved elusive. At the foundations, it was not until the middle of the program that its co-funders were able to agree upon a collaborative oversight arrangement.

Although the initiative did not bring about the hoped-for results, it did leave some long-lasting benefits behind in the participating communities. More than half of the sites were considered either exemplary in preparing students for the health professions or having developed excellent components, such as teacher training programs, quality after-school, weekend, and summer enrichment programs, and strong partnerships between community organization and schools.[17] Even programs that do not achieve their overall goals can have positive effects on the people they touch.

—⚡— Programs that Did Not Meet Expectations Because of a Challenging or Changing Environment

It is ironic that the areas of highest priority for the Foundation— areas such as expanding health insurance coverage, improving quality, and reducing childhood obesity—are precisely those that are most difficult to affect because they face the greatest societal challenges. SUPPORT, the Generalist Physician Initiative, and Strengthening Hospital Nursing are programs that were designed to bring about change in areas that the Foundation considered as priorities. All three ran into social, political, or economic barriers that led to disappointing results.

SUPPORT

SUPPORT, the Study to Understand Prognoses and Preferences for Outcomes and Risks of Treatment, a $31 million research project that the Robert Wood Johnson Foundation funded between 1988 and 1996, did not achieve the result that the Foundation had hoped for: improving the care of dying hospitalized patients. The program trained teams of nurses whose job it was to communicate patients' wishes for treatment (or withholding of treatment) to physicians and then to work with family members and physicians to see that those wishes were carried out. A rigorous evaluation found that the program led to absolutely no improvement.[18]

Neither doctors nor hospitals nor nurses nor patients nor their families were able to overcome the inertia of the system.

Despite the attention to end-of-life care from high-profile legal cases, the publicity given to living wills, and SUPPORT itself, end-of-life care did not improve. As SUPPORT's co-principal investigator, Joanne Lynn, wrote, "Physicians did not know what patients wanted with regard to resuscitation, even though these patients were at high risk of cardiac arrest. . . . Most patients who died in the hospital spent most of their last days on ventilators in intensive care." Except for the comatose, Lynn noted, more than half of the patients were reported to have substantial pain.[19]

What makes SUPPORT so instructive is the Robert Wood Johnson Foundation's reaction to these discouraging results. Faced with an intervention that achieved so little, the Foundation developed a whole new end-of-life program area out of SUPPORT's ashes. Steven Schroeder, the president of the Robert Wood Johnson Foundation at the time, recalled, "One of the program officers behind SUPPORT came into my office, practically in tears that the program had not worked. My reaction was, 'Let's take this lemon and make the most delicious lemonade out of it that anybody has tasted.'"

The Foundation developed its recipe for lemonade by embarking on an ambitious $170 million effort between 1996 and 2005 to improve the care given to dying patients—one that, in combination with the work of the Open Society Institute, knowledgeable observers credit with building a field of palliative care in the United States, even though it is still not known whether the care of dying patients has in fact improved.

The Generalist Physician Initiative

Since its very first days, the Robert Wood Johnson Foundation has been trying to restructure the medical care system from one built around specialists to one built around primary care practitioners. The Foundation's interest in primary care—or generalist medicine, as it is sometimes called—has continued through the decades. Nonetheless, interest among medical students in careers as generalists had declined throughout the 1980s, reaching its nadir in 1992, when fewer than 15 percent of medical school graduates planned careers in primary care (down from 36 percent in 1982).

To attract more medical students to careers in primary care, the Foundation launched a $100 million cluster of programs in the early 1990s. The centerpiece was the Generalist Physician Initiative, a seven-year, $33 million program. It was designed to influence four points considered critical to attracting medical students to careers as generalist physicians (that is, as general internists, general pediatricians, and family practitioners). The four points were admissions, undergraduate medical curriculum, residency programs, and setting up practice. The fifteen medical schools that administered the Generalist Physician Initiative did, in fact, address each of these points by, for example, marketing themselves as generalist schools, changing the admissions process to target more students with generalist potential, adding generalists to admissions committees, introducing primary care into the curriculum at an early stage, creating more primary care residency slots, and forgiving loans to students choosing primary care practice.

Enrollment in generalist tracks at the participating schools did increase somewhat, but no more than in the nonparticipating medical schools. In the mid- and late-1990s, there was a brief surge in interest in generalist careers as medical school students responded to managed care companies' need for primary care physicians as entry points in the system and gatekeepers.[20] So enrollment in generalist tracks increased across the board.

After the backlash against managed care led to reducing the role of generalist physicians and strengthening that of specialists, the percentages of medical students seeking primary care slots sank again. Between 1997 and 2002, for example, the number of American medical school graduates in family practice residencies declined by 19 percent. Joel Klompus, a San Francisco-based physician and president of the board of directors of Brown & Toland, a large physicians' group in California, commented, "It has become almost impossible to attract medical students to careers in primary care. There are so many incentives driving them into specialties."

In retrospect, the Generalist Physician Initiative was a worthy but unsuccessful endeavor. It bestowed the Foundation's imprimatur on an issue that the Foundation considered important, much as the Foundation's work to expand health insurance coverage and increase the percentage of minority health practitioners—equally challenging assignments—give a certain credibility to these issues. It did not, however, change either the culture of medical schools, the aspirations of medical students, or the number of primary care physicians. Foundations do not have the power to change the economic climate in which career decisions are made. Given a reimbursement system favoring specialty care and the high prestige of specialists (compared with the heavy workload and comparatively low income of primary care physicians), it is little wonder that medical students are not clamoring to become generalist physicians. As the deputy director of the Generalist Physician Initiative, Gerald Perkoff, a physician and, at the time, professor at the University of Missouri Medical School, wrote, "Market forces have more to do with career choice than do the needs of the system, and certainly more than philosophies."[21]

Strengthening Hospital Nursing

The Strengthening Hospital Nursing Program did not meet expectations, but for somewhat different reasons than the examples discussed above; the circumstances under which the program was planned changed markedly as the program was being implemented, rendering the original objectives difficult to reach.

In the late 1980s, as the Strengthening Hospital Nursing Program was being conceived, the country was in the midst of a nursing shortage. Among the reasons cited for the nursing shortage was a high level of job dissatisfaction. To address this, the Robert Wood Johnson Foundation, in collaboration with The Pew Charitable Trusts, developed a program to make hospital nursing a more attractive profession. The program had a second goal, improving patient care. Thus the full title of the program—Strengthening Hospital Nursing: A Program to Improve Patient Care.

The two goals were not necessarily compatible. As the program developed, the second goal was interpreted quite broadly to mean a restructuring of the way hospitals were run. "The Strengthening Hospital Nursing Program seeks to bring about a fundamental change in the US hospital," Barbara Donaho and Mary Kay Kohles, the program's director and deputy director, wrote.[22] Mitchell Rabkin, at the time the president of Beth Israel Hospital, a grantee of the program, viewed the kind of change envisioned by the program as one recognizing "that the hospital is fundamentally a nursing institution." [23]

Between 1990 and 1995, twelve hospitals and eight hospital consortia participated in the Strengthening Hospital Nursing Program. Each grantee had considerable flexibility about how to structure its $1 million implementation grant, and each took a somewhat different route.

Despite improvements in some of the participating hospitals, characterized by the evaluation team from the University of California, Berkeley, as running "deep and wide," the program was overtaken by the changing health care workforce.[24] Even as the program was ramping up, the nursing shortage was disappearing. Managed care companies, which came to dominate health care in the 1990s, were laying off nurses and looking for less well-trained personnel to fill their roles. With nurses fearing for their jobs, they were hardly in a position to demand that hospital care be organized around them.

Strengthening Hospital Nursing appears to have had positive results in some of the hospitals in the program.[25] Viewed from a broad perspective, however, the program neither succeeded in restructuring hospital care around nursing nor in improving patient care. Making this kind of systemic change is difficult in any environment, and even more so in one in which managed care made the position of hospital nurses so tenuous. As the program's evaluators concluded, "The importance of larger economic forces on hospital decision making cannot be ignored."[26]

Both the Strengthening Hospital Nursing Program and the Generalist Physician Initiative underscore the need to keep track of the social, political, and economic environment in which programs operate, and to make programmatic revisions that may be required by changing circumstances.

—⚬— Programs that Did Not Meet Expectations Primarily Because of Faulty Execution

Programs sometimes do not work out because they are poorly managed, because the leadership is flawed, because they unnecessarily deviate from the original plan, or for the many reasons that implementation suffers. In any given case, flawed execution can trump even the best-planned strategy. "After observing many organizations, including the Robert Wood Johnson Foundation, I think that foundations tend to overemphasize strategy at the expense of execution," wrote Steven Schroeder.[27] The Clinical Nurse Scholars Program and the Center for Child Well-being offer examples of programs whose lack of success was attributable primarily to flawed execution.

The Clinical Nurse Scholars Program

At the time of the nursing shortage of the early 1980s, staff members at the Robert Wood Johnson Foundation identified a problem: nursing schools were graduating nurses who had strong academic backgrounds but were unprepared for the real world of hospital nursing. "Nurses started their careers in a sort of culture shock because they weren't prepared," noted

Carolyn Newbergh, a health writer.[28] To address this problem, the Foundation developed the Clinical Nurse Scholars Program to train a core of nursing professors and leaders who would reorient academic nursing around clinical skills. Modeled on what was considered the Foundation's signature program, the Clinical Scholars Program for physicians, the Clinical Nurse Scholars Program began in 1982 and, with extensions, was expected to run through 1994. Carried out in three of the nation's leading nursing schools—the University of California, San Francisco, the University of Pennsylvania, and the University of Rochester—the program was to provide two years of training to nine nursing faculty members a year.

A Foundation review of the program completed in 1987 concluded that the program had deviated from its objective. Rather than emphasizing clinical teaching skills, it had become a vehicle to finance the doctoral studies of clinical nurse scholars and, in addition, was no longer focused on hospital nursing. The Foundation's leadership was so upset with the direction the program had taken that it ended the program early, funding seven classes instead of the ten that had been originally planned.

In succeeding years, a consensus has developed that this decision was an overly drastic response to a genuine problem of program execution. The former president and executive vice-president of the Foundation (along with one of the co-authors of this chapter, Stephen Isaacs), concluded in 1997, "The Clinical Nurse Scholars Program probably was terminated prematurely; although it had veered from its original objectives, it might have been redesigned to overcome some of its problems." Nor did the Foundation act in partnership with its grantees, or even listen to them. According to Newbergh, those involved in the program, who have since become leaders of academic nursing, felt that "[the Foundation] didn't understand that for nurses to gain prominence as leaders, they needed to follow the same path as the nation's most noted doctors—by developing expertise in research."[29]

The Clinical Nurse Scholars Program illustrates the need for regular program monitoring so that deviations from original objectives can be identified early, as well as the need to carefully consider drastic steps, such as premature closure of a program, before taking them. Ironically, in the face of a more recent nursing shortage, in 2008, the Foundation issued a call for proposals for a new program called the Robert Wood Johnson Foundation Nurse Faculty Scholars whose objective, "to help talented junior nursing faculty advance in their careers by giving them the opportunity to develop a research program and participate in other scholarly activities,"[30] is almost identical to the one that had led to the Clinical Nurse Scholars Program's termination nearly twenty years earlier.

The Center for Child Well-being

In response to a board directive, in mid-1996 the Foundation created an internal task force to explore what more it could do to improve children's health. One recommendation to emerge from the task force was the establishment of a new center that would, among its other roles, be a major force in disseminating objective, scientifically sound information on child health and development and play a leading role in advancing children's health nationally. The Foundation invited William Foege, a physician and one of the giants in public health, to develop and head the center, an invitation he accepted only after considerable arm-twisting, according to former Foundation senior vice-president Ruby Hearn.

Foege submitted an ambitious proposal, a scaled-down version of which the Foundation funded in February 1999. Under the $9 million grant, the Atlanta-based Task Force for Child Survival and Development, headed by Foege, would set up a new Center for Child Well-being whose work would include using a scientific approach to identify each of the critical elements of healthy development for children, adopting sophisticated communications strategies to translate what had been learned from research into practice, and strengthening leadership within the child health and development community. Foege became director of the center on a half-time basis.[31]

Roughly seven months after the proposal was funded, Foege accepted a position as a senior adviser to the emerging Bill & Melinda Gates Foundation, allowing him to return to his first passion, global health. A few months later, his deputy resigned for unrelated personal reasons. Although Foege remained the Center's executive director at the agreed-upon 50 percent level and the deputy was replaced, Foundation staff members felt that there was a leadership vacuum at the top.

Partly because of this, and partly because the center had not met some of the benchmarks that had been established (for example, developing a Web site, establishing a virtual network of collaborators, and forging relations with other children's health groups), a proposal for expanding the Center, submitted in late 2000, ran into tough sledding at the Foundation. Staff members pointed out that the Center had made limited progress on some of its key benchmarks. As Paul Jellinek, a Foundation vice president at the time and currently a private consultant, observed, "We never had a clear understanding of what it added up to." The result: instead of supporting the Center at an increased level for three years, as requested, the Foundation agreed to only eighteen months' funding, after which the Center would be on its own. Currently, the Center is still connected with the Task Force for Child Survival and Development, and has a Web site.

—⬥— Learning from Programs that Haven't Met Expectations

Increasingly, foundations are attempting to establish clear goals and measurable strategies, assess progress against them, and, most important, learn from their successes and failures. Every program is different, however, and provides lessons that may be applicable only to its own situation. It is hard to compare a tobacco-control program, for example, with one to improve the care of chronically ill patients. Even so, some general lessons emerge from this review of programs that have not met expectations.

Managing Expectations

In a two-trillion-dollar-plus health economy with political, social, and economic factors that often seem beyond anyone's control, one cannot realistically expect a single program—or even a cluster of programs—to bring about major social change. The political, social, and economic barriers faced by social-change programs—such as those to expand generalist medicine, increase health insurance coverage, reduce obesity, and improve quality of care—are enormous. But fostering social change is exactly what big foundations such as Robert Wood Johnson often aim to do.

A first lesson to emerge from the analysis of programs that did not meet expectations is that major foundations ought to address important issues and enunciate ambitious goals of changing social policy but that expectations for success should be tempered. In the words of Joel Fleishman, currently a Duke University professor and one of the leading thinkers on foundation accountability, foundations should "recognize that a bit of humility is appropriate when grappling with major social change."[32] Unfortunately, many foundation staff members are tempted to oversell a program to get its approval.

How much humility? There is no simple formula to guide how much risk of failure a foundation should be prepared to accept. Fleishman observed, "For-profit venture capitalists...expect eight or nine of every ten investments to fail, and one or two to succeed mightily."[33] While such a low success rate may be hard to swallow in philanthropy, a tolerance for lack of success must be built into programs that attempt to bring about social change. As The Hewlett Foundation's Paul Brest observed, "If nothing seems to be working, then one must reconsider the goal and the strategies of reaching it. And it makes sense to set intermediate targets that get measured along the way. If short-term and intermediate-term targets are not being met, it is unlikely that the long-term goals will be."

Moreover, programs may gradually chip away at the problem in ways that cannot be easily seen until something happens outside the control of the foundation, such as a new law or policy. To take an example from another foundation, The California Endowment worked for years to promote policies that would ban the sale of junk food and soda in the state's public schools, without visible success. Almost overnight the political situation changed. A new governor interested in halting childhood obesity was elected, and the state legislature passed laws banning junk food and soda from being sold in the state's public schools.[34]

The staff and the board of the Robert Wood Johnson Foundation have grappled with questions of risk and expectations. Risa Lavizzo-Mourey, the president and CEO of the Robert Wood Johnson Foundation, noted that "the trustees have given the staff a lot of leeway to tackle big problems such as childhood obesity and quality of care, to adopt bold approaches, and even to fail if they don't work out. There are no constraints placed on us because a program might fail or even embarrass us."

Clarifying Objectives and Strategies

In a recent study of business failure, Paul Carroll and Chunka Mui concluded that most avoidable failures are due to flawed strategies.[35] Although foundations don't have to meet the same bottom line as businesses do, they have a bottom line to meet nonetheless. According to Phil Buchanan, the president of The Center for Effective Philanthropy, "People don't define goals and strategies well enough. So they can't know what works and what doesn't."

This is the case in some of the programs examined above. In the Strengthening Hospital Nursing Program, it was unclear whether the objective was to strengthen the practice of nursing in hospitals or to restructure the way hospitals were administered. In the Health Professions Partnership Initiative, the intervention was not robust enough to lead to the desired result. In the National Health Care Purchasing Institute, discussed in chapter 3, it was not clear whether the program was aimed at the public sector, the private sector, or both.

Since 2003, the Robert Wood Johnson Foundation has been using an "impact framework" that sets out and guides the board, the staff, and the grantees in short-, medium-, and long-term objectives.[36] "Laying out a framework for people in the field—the ones doing the work—that gives them the ability to know how they are doing is critical," Lavizzo-Mourey said. "It also gives them the ability to know where they are and to know that no program is likely to be 100 percent successful or 100 percent failure."

Focusing on Goals but Remaining Strategically Flexible

Pierre Omidyar, the founder of eBay, in a speech to the 2002 graduating class at Tufts University, said, "Prepare for the unexpected...Sometimes ideas have ideas of their own...In the deepest sense, eBay wasn't a hobby. And it wasn't a business. It was—and is—a community: an organic, evolving, self-organizing web of individual relationships, formed around shared interests."[37]

"Prepare for the unexpected!" For philanthropy, the lesson is: remain flexible enough to alter tactics while not losing sight of the overall goal. As Tony Proscio observes in chapter 2 of this volume, several Foundation-funded programs went through midcourse corrections after it became clear that the original plans were not working.

A related point is not to be wedded to strategies that aren't effective in practice. Former president Steven Schroeder, looking back at the Foundation's efforts to build community coalitions, observed, "I am not sure that our logic model was correct. I don't think there was evidence that you could mobilize communities absent already existing coalitions, which often start with a group of committed advocates, such as breast cancer advocates.... After a while, the formation of coalitions itself became the goal rather than a strategy to reach the intended goal."

Monitoring and Assessing Programs

For the most part, program officers at foundations are motivated largely by the development of new and exciting programs. Once a program is conceived and approved, it is easy to forget it and move on to the next. Evaluation is often left for the very end, and in too many cases is an afterthought. One lesson from this review is the importance of routine monitoring of programs, including the social-economic-political context in which they are developing, and acting upon reports of changed circumstances. The recession of 2008–2009 offers a telling example. "When state budgets went south with the deteriorating economy, our programs struggled," Lavizzo-Mourey said. "We have to be prepared to react quickly to external circumstances like those."

Related to that is the importance of incorporating evaluation very early in the life of a program. Supporting Families After Welfare Reform, discussed in chapter 2, is an example of a program where monitoring and listening early to the problems expressed by grantees led to a restructuring that probably saved it. The Health Professions Partnership Initiative and Best Friends are examples of programs where an evaluation (or in the case of Best Friends, the prospect of an evaluation) came too late to address fundamental flaws that, had they been disclosed earlier, might have been remedied.

The development of formal logic models specifying the theory of change for an individual program or a cluster of programs and the identification of indicators of major events or outcomes are useful tools to monitor developments, and the Foundation has utilized them since the late 1990s.[38] Yet even they do not provide a full understanding of strategies undertaken by the Foundation. A third point relating to monitoring and assessment to emerge from this review is the importance of reviewing entire strategies, not just programs or clusters of programs, at a mid-way point.

—ᴧᴧ— Dealing with Programs that Don't Meet Expectations

There are a number of ways of dealing with programs that do not work out as planned. The most dramatic example of turning around a disappointment is SUPPORT, where the failure of the intervention led to a major new effort to improve end-of-life care. In other cases, such as the SmokeLess States program and the Supporting Families After Welfare Reform (discussed in chapter 2), programs underwent a midcourse correction after it became clear that the planned approaches were not working. For the most part, however, ineffective programs simply continue until the grant period is over.

There does come a time, however, when a program has such troubles that it cannot be saved, even if modified, and the Foundation should pull the plug. This happened with Community Programs for Affordable Health Care, the Center for Child Well-being, and the National Institute for Health Care Purchasing Institute (discussed in chapter 3). The Clinical Nurse Scholars Program was also terminated early, though in retrospect, the termination appears to have been premature.

Since every program is different, each will require a decision appropriate to the particular circumstances. As a rule, unless a program goes completely off in a wrong direction, the wise course is for the Foundation and grantees to work together to try to correct it. The Foundation considers that it is in a collaborative relationship with its grantees and that both are working for the common good. As such, problems that arise are considered to be common ones that both the grantee and the Foundation should try to resolve in partnership. "Ideally, the Foundation and its grantees will have developed a relationship as partners and will have the openness and flexibility to fix problems, even major ones, as they develop," Risa Lavizzo-Mourey said in a recent interview.

—ᴡᴡ— Conclusion

The Robert Wood Johnson Foundation is widely considered as being in the forefront of learning from its programmatic experiences and, through vehicles such as published program evaluations, its Grant Results Reports, which are posted on the Foundation's Web site, and this *Anthology* series, sharing what it has learned. The Foundation is striving to develop a culture whereby the staff and the board learn from the results of its programs, both positive and negative, though Foundation staff members candidly confess that there is a long way to go.

We have chosen to avoid the word "failure," since even programs that do not work as expected can provide valuable lessons and directions for the future. SUPPORT led to a twenty-year effort to address problems in end-of- life care. Health Link, a prisoner re-entry program, had no significant effects on recidivism, but influenced the field's approach to re-entry.[39] Failure occurs when lessons are not learned or communicated to others.

More foundations are attempting to be strategic in their grant making, scrutinizing the results of their programs more carefully, and even making their successes and failures public. The James Irvine Foundation, for example, posted a case study of a program that underwent a midcourse correction on its Web site. For the past twelve years, The Wallace Foundation has posted all of its program evaluations—positive and negative—on its Web site. "Though we encounter sensitivities and concerns, the effects have been positive," said Ed Pauly, the director of evaluation at The Wallace Foundation. "The program staff, in particular, finds the posted evaluations very useful and uses evidence about programs that have not worked out as a way of improving future programs." And The Hewlett Foundation posts the results of The Center for Effective Philanthropy's surveys about the foundation.

Yet, at this point, there is more talk than action. "There is a great rhetorical embrace of being strategic, adopting performance indicators, and measuring results," The Center for Effective Philanthropy's Phil Buchanan said. "However, there is still a big gap between the rhetoric and what people actually do."

Even though action lags behind words, there is clearly some momentum in philanthropy toward understanding impact, reporting on results (even negative results), and sharing them with the field when appropriate. Who knows, maybe in the not-too-distant future, it will become the norm.

Notes

1. Newbergh, C. "The Robert Wood Johnson Foundation's Efforts to Contain Health Care Costs." *To Improve Health and Health Care: The Robert Wood Johnson Foundation Anthology, Vol. VII.* San Francisco: Jossey-Bass, 2004.
2. Brown, L. D., and McLaughlin, C. "Constraining Costs at the Community Level: A Critique." *Health Affairs*, 9(4), 1990, 5–28.
3. Cohen, A. B., Cantor, J. C., and Schroeder, S. A. "Perspectives: The Funders." *Health Affairs*, 9(4), 1990, 29–33.
4. Stiles, G. M., and Dunlop, J. T. "Perspectives: A Local Program and a National Advisory Chairman." *Health Affairs*, 9(4), 1990, 42–46.
5. Cohodes, D. R. "Perspectives: A Private Insurer." *Health Affairs*, 9 (4), 1990, 34–37.
6. Brown and McLaughlin, "Constraining Costs at the Community Level."
7. The program, which was for girls at the time the Robert Wood Johnson Foundation funded it, was later expanded to include boys and high schools.
8. Bennett, E. Best Friends Foundation, http://www.bestfriendsfoundation.org. Accessed on June 6, 2009.
9. The National Campaign to Prevent Teen Pregnancy, http://www.thenationalcampaign.org/policymakers/PDF/abstinence_04_07.pdf. Accessed on June 6, 2009.
10. The Foundation also provided separate support to a Best Friends program in a Newark, New Jersey, high school, initially through the New Jersey Health Initiatives program.

11. Mathematica Policy Research. *Impacts of Four Title V, Section 510 Abstinence Education Programs: Final Report*, April 2007. The evaluation concluded: "Findings indicate that youth in the program were no more likely than the control group to have abstained from sex and, among those who reported having sex, they had similar numbers of sexual partners and had initiated sex at the same mean age."

12. Carline, J. D., and Patterson, D. G. "Characteristics of Health Professions Schools, Public School Systems, and Community-Based Organizations in Successful Partnerships to Increase the Numbers of Underrepresented Minority Students Entering Health Professions Education." *Academic Medicine*, 81, 2006, S2–4.

13. Ibid.

14. Cleveland, E. F. "Telling the Stories of the Health Professions Partnership Initiative." *Academic Medicine*, 81 (6 Syppl), 2006, S15–16.

15. Carline and Patterson.

16. Terrell C. "Foreword: The Health Professions Partnership Initiative and Working Towards Diversity in the Health Care Workforce." *Academic Medicine*, 81 (6 Syppl), 2006, S2–4.

17. Ibid.

18. Schroeder, S. A. "The Legacy of Support Study to Understand Prognosis and Preferences for Outcomes and Risks of Treatment." *Annals of Internal Medicine*, 131(10), 1999, 780–782; Weisfeld, V., Miller, D., Gibon, R. and Schroeder, S. A. "Improving Care at the End of Life: What Does It Take?" *Health Affairs*, 19(6), 2000, 277–283.

19. Lynn, J. "Unexpected Returns: Insights from SUPPORT." *To Improve Health and Health Care: The Robert Wood Johnson Foundation Anthology, 1997*. San Francisco: Jossey-Bass, 1997.

20. Colwill, J. M. "Primary Care Medicine and the Education of Generalist Physicians: Past, Present and Future." *Generalist Medicine*. San Francisco: Jossey Bass, 2004, p. 24.

21. The Robert Wood Johnson Foundation. "The Generalist Physicians Initiative." *Grants Results Report*, July 22, 2003. http://www.rwjf.org/pr/product.jsp?id=17971. Accessed on June 6, 2009.

22. Quoted in Rundall, T. G., Starkweather, D. B., and Norrish, B. "The Strengthening Hospital Nursing Program." *To Improve Health and Health Care: The Robert Wood Johnson Foundation, 1998–1999*. San Francisco: Jossey-Bass, 1999.

23. Rundall, T. G., Starkweather, D. B., and Norrish, B. "The Strengthening Hospital Nursing Program." *To Improve Health and Health Care: The Robert Wood Johnson Foundation, 1998–1999*. San Francisco: Jossey-Bass, 1999.

24. Ibid.

25. Ibid.

26. Ibid.
27. Schroeder, S. A. "When Execution Trumps Strategy." *Just Money: A Critique of Contemporary American Philanthropy*, Karoff, H. P., ed. Boston: TPI Editions, 2004, p. 185.
28. Newbergh, C. "The RWJF Commitment to Nursing." *To Improve Health and Health Care: The Robert Wood Johnson Foundation Anthology, Vol. VIII*. San Francisco: Jossey-Bass, 2005.
29. Ibid.
30. The Robert Wood Johnson Foundation. "RWJF Awards Fifteen Nurse Faculty Scholars Research and Mentoring Support." *News Release*. www.rwjf.org/pr/product.jsp?id=34429. Accessed on June 6, 2009.
31. The Robert Wood Johnson Foundation. "Center Goes National to Solve Children's Health Issues but Ends Up Local." *Grant Results Report*, 2003. www.rwjf.org/reports/grr/040325.htm. Accessed on June 6, 2009.
32. Fleishman, J. L. "Simply Doing Good or Doing Good Well: Stewardship, Hubris, and Foundation Governance." *Just Money: A Critique of Contemporary American Philanthropy*, Karoff, H. P., ed. Boston: TPI Editions, 2004, p. 107.
33. Ibid.
34. Isaacs, S. L., and Swartz, A. *Junk Food and Soda Sales in the Public Schools*. The California Endowment, 2006.
35. Carroll, P. B., and Mui, C. "7 Ways to Fail Big: Lessons from the Most Inexcusable Failures of the Past 25 Years." *Harvard Business Review*, September 2008, 82–91.
36. See Lavizzo-Mourey, R. "Foreword." *To Improve Health and Health Care: The Robert Wood Johnson Foundation Anthology, Vol. VII*. San Francisco: Jossey-Bass, 2004, for a discussion of the impact framework.
37. Quoted by Karoff in *Just Money: A Critique of Contemporary American Philanthropy*, Karoff, H. P., ed. Boston: TPI Editions, 2004, p. 17.
38. See Knickman, J. R., and Hunt, K. A. "The Robert Wood Johnson Foundation's Approach to Evaluation." *To Improve Health and Health Policy: The Robert Wood Johnson Foundation, Vol. XI*. San Francisco: Jossey-Bass, 2008.
39. See Bunch, W. "Helping Former Prisoners Reenter Society: The Health Link Project." *To Improve Health and Health Policy: The Robert Wood Johnson Foundation Anthology, Vol. XII*. San Francisco: Jossey-Bass, 2009.

CHAPTER 2

New Direction, Midcourse: Redesigning a Program While It's in Progress

Tony Proscio

—ɯ— **W**hen foundations place big strategic bets on long-term programs, allocating millions of dollars for years of effort, the choice of a basic strategy can be a bit like building a railroad. Painstaking work and major capital investment go into laying the track and lining up the moving equipment—after which the course is largely set. Yes, the engines can be upgraded, new cars can be added, and, as Amtrak proved, higher-speed trains can even be mounted on old lines. But the fundamental route—in foundation terms, the strategic outlines—can be changed only with difficulty, expense, and disruption. In practice, such changes are rare.

Mapping a strategy for a major philanthropic program involves dozens of early decisions that are meant to hold firm for four, five, even ten years into the future. For example, at the

Robert Wood Johnson Foundation, large programs are typically managed by a national program office, chosen at the beginning of a program's life. The national program office is usually a separate organization (or part of a larger organization) charged with over-seeing and administering the Foundation's grants and providing expert assistance to grantees year after year. The selection of a national program office consequently determines a lot about the program's substance and style: how it will work with grantees and their collaborators, what kinds of expertise will be brought to bear in what ways, how the program's lessons and message will be presented to the wider world, and much more.

Further, by the time the national program office starts its work, many other decisions with long-term consequences have been made: Overall strategies have been developed; the board has authorized an amount for the program; expectations of grantees have been carefully reviewed and committed to paper; and means of measuring progress and gauging success or failure have often been set in motion. All these decisions can be altered later, of course. But like relaying a railroad track, those later changes are apt to be difficult and expensive.

Most of the time, this relative inflexibility is a necessity, even a virtue. Many foundation programs set out to test ideas whose merits will take years to prove, and are sure to encounter surprises and rough spots along the way. Patience and perseverance are supposed to be hallmarks of strategic philanthropy for precisely this reason. Changing course too soon can deprive a good idea of the time and backing it needs to accumulate resources, win allies, and overcome obstacles.

Even beyond these strategic considerations, changing course can have human costs that aren't always apparent or frankly acknowledged. For starters, big foundation programs are usually the product of months, even years, of research, thought, and planning by some of the foundation's more distinguished officers and the experts with whom they consult. Their reputations, and the fate of ideas in which they believe strongly, are on the line when a new program launches. A decision to amend the plan later will usually require that the same people who gave birth to it, advocated for it, and managed its early development now have to acknowledge that it isn't quite what they had envisioned. That acknowledgment can, in some cases, affect their reputations as well as their hope of making an important breakthrough in their field. Grantee organizations, in turn, will have hired staff, bought equipment, perhaps rented space, and staked their own reputations on implementing the original plan. A midcourse change may reflect poorly on their work, or may even result in reduced grant support, terminated jobs, and strained relations with other participants in the program.

Michael Rothman, a senior program officer at the Robert Wood Johnson Foundation from 1998 to 2004, experienced this mix of strategic and human pressures firsthand. "Usually a program is pretty personal to a program officer," he says. "There's usually one main person behind it, and no one else is watching the events as carefully, or has so much invested in it. So [as a program officer] you're always the advocate for your program, and you tend to see things as going well even if they aren't." For all these reasons, he concludes, "programs tend to be pretty linear. The Foundation gives you money for a period of time, and you're on that path. Programs aren't designed to be changed along the way."

As a result, midcourse corrections often come about when new personnel arrive on the scene. Risa Lavizzo-Mourey, the Robert Wood Johnson Foundation's president and chief executive officer, notes that "a shift in program staff makes it possible to view a program through a different lens." New officers "may see things that staff working on a program for years might have overlooked, or they might just see the opportunities and context a little differently." Yet even then, she adds, the tendency is usually to make tactical adjustments or shift priorities among existing elements of the program, not to disrupt the elementary strategy on which the initiative is based.

Still, the need for fundamental change is sometimes inescapable, and the rail line has to be rerouted. Although the reasons for this aren't always negative, the consequences nearly always involve difficult, often uncomfortable changes in the lives of a program's key personnel.

—⟶⟵— Three Reasons for Changing Course

Changes in strategy can arise for any number of reasons, but the most common causes for a midcourse correction tend to fall into three categories. The first of these may have little or nothing to do with the strategy itself: sometimes events and circumstances simply overwhelm the best-laid plans. Markets or the political climate may turn sharply more hospitable to the program's intent—or more hostile. Advances in technology or research may bring a sudden boost or bust. Opportunity or obstacles may surface from unexpected quarters: a celebrity or an ultrawealthy donor suddenly takes up the cause; a news event galvanizes public interest; or the program stumbles onto an idea that produces unexpectedly explosive results.

Even in the happiest of these cases, an unexpected change in the environment can impose serious new costs and disruptions: If the environment becomes dramatically more fertile or the program encounters far more opportunity than expected, the model may then have to be retooled for major growth. Worse, the growth opportunities often arise not in the whole program as originally designed but only in certain parts of it. In that case, the course correction may well involve paring back the less successful elements and concentrating support on those that have the greatest potential. Some activities (and maybe some grantees) will lose money and stature, or even shut down entirely. In short, there can be disruptions and disappointments even when changes derive from unexpected opportunity and lead to accelerated growth.

In a second category of midcourse corrections are programs whose strategy was never quite right in the first place. As the work begins to unfold, cracks in the model become more apparent: assumptions that don't match reality, forecasts about budgets and workloads that prove unrealistic, expected allies and resources that never materialize, partners and beneficiaries who don't behave as predicted. These can be the hardest cases for the program's designers, who now have to combat the twin temptations of human nature in confronting error: denying the problem and blaming other people. Even assuming that they face the problem forthrightly and devise a smart alternative plan, their proposals for saving the program will run into headwinds of doubt and anxiety that always gather strength whenever disappointment is in the air.

A third category of course correction can be even touchier: when a program's underlying model may be fine but the execution is falling short. In this case, it's the implementers, more than the designers, who must bear the brunt of the failure and disappointment. Admittedly, cases of this sort can be hard to diagnose precisely. As Steven Schroeder, president of the Robert Wood Johnson Foundation from 1990 to 2002, points out, when implementation is flawed, "the only thing you can say is that, but for the execution, the model *might* have worked—but we will never know."

Amid the uncertainty, the mounting disagreements between designers and implementers, grant makers and grant recipients, can become painful, involving exchanges of blame, disputes over the meaning of past agreements, even clashes of values. These tensions can grow even more difficult when the perceived shortcomings are ascribed to implementers who are otherwise valued allies, performing with distinction on other work for the Foundation and other funders. In that case, the potential for ill feeling and mistrust can have ripple effects beyond the program being redesigned.

In the next few pages, we consider examples of each type of course correction and see how Foundation officers diagnosed the problem, reconsidered their initial strategy, and worked with national program directors and others involved in the program to set a new direction. Two of the examples involve programs that the Foundation funded and that are discussed by name. In the case of programs that suffered from flawed implementation, however, it is necessary to create a composite of programs that actually occurred, but where the activities that took place and the identities of the people who directed the programs are disguised. This is because in those cases, the best examples involved disappointments and disagreements that were partly personal and are still raw. The cases involve people who, despite their disagreements, have too much regard for one another to be willing to air disparaging information in print. The result is an accurate description of problems and choices, bolstered by unaltered comments of actual participants, but presented in a way that isn't traceable to specific people and events.

Two on-the-record cases involve retooling to meet changed conditions and repairing a flawed strategy. The first involves SmokeLess States, a tobacco-control program that was significantly expanded in midcourse, and the second describes Supporting Families After Welfare Reform, a program to extend health benefits to more low-income families, which was re-engineered when some of its initial assumptions proved wrong. The third, composite case, describes what happened when the Foundation felt it had to change the way a program was being implemented—and some of the people who were implementing it.

—⟋⟋— Overtaken by Events: Adapting a Program to New Circumstances

In 1993, the Robert Wood Johnson Foundation launched a $10 million program to reduce smoking and raise public awareness of the health benefits of quitting tobacco. The new program, called SmokeLess States, was at first based on a general belief that coalitions of medical and public health organizations, working in concert, would be an effective voice for reducing smoking and promoting tobacco-control policies in states and localities. The coalitions typically included local chapters of the American Heart Association, the American Lung Association, and the American Cancer Society, plus health care organizations and medical societies.

The theory was still partly inchoate when the first nineteen grants were made, in 1994. Envisioning only a small demonstration, program designers set out mainly to see how much potential the idea might have. As the Foundation's interest in tobacco control rose throughout the 1990s, the program grew to thirty states with a supplemental allocation of $20 million in 1996. Even then, the strategic aims of SmokeLess States remained broad and malleable, encompassing public education, programs to discourage smoking, and advocacy for tobacco-control policies, such as increased excise taxes and clean indoor air ordinances, at the state and local levels. Work across the thirty sites varied widely, depending on the strength, the experience, and the interests of the coalitions in each place.

Some coalitions were being formed from scratch, and therefore spent many months simply getting organized and learning to deliberate as a group. Among those that launched programs, many chose fairly traditional public health activities meant to discourage smoking, like youth education activities, programs in schools, and public service ads. Groups tended to spread their resources among several lines of work rather than concentrating on one or two main goals.

In the original design of SmokeLess States, policy change had been just one of several activities the project directors were encouraged to consider, although Nancy Kaufman, a former Foundation vice president who was an architect of the program, had encouraged policy work from the beginning. A few pioneering state coalitions took up Kaufman's challenge and used the Foundation grants and other funds for vigorous, well-focused campaigns to make far-reaching change in public policy. Coalitions in Alaska and Hawaii quickly launched successful efforts to raise cigarette taxes, as did Arizona soon thereafter. These early efforts suggested how much might be possible if more coalitions made a disciplined, deliberate effort on the policy front.

New research was making the case for changing public policy even stronger. Alongside SmokeLess States, the Foundation had created the Tobacco Policy Research and Evaluation Program specifically aimed at measuring the health effects of various tobacco laws and regulations. More and more, findings from that program were pointing to two clear leaders in reducing smoking-related disease among young people: cigarette taxes and clean-indoor-air laws, each of which had been pushed by one or more SmokeLess States coalitions.

By the end of the program's fourth year, it was clear that many activities funded under SmokeLess States were too small and diffuse to lead to any significant reductions in youth smoking. The exception was the legislative work. But in how many states could such work succeed? And, given the fierce resistance of the tobacco industry and its political allies, was the Foundation prepared to mount a policy effort large enough, and deliberate enough, to make a difference? "Passing a tax increase or a clean-indoor-air law isn't a one-time dance," Kaufman points out. "You need several legislative sessions to do this. You need to marshal your research and public education, hone your message, demonstrate public support. And then you need time to make that message stick." Could the Foundation support enough states, for enough time, to propel a national bandwagon to raise taxes and enact clean-indoor-air laws?

Fortunately, by this time the ground was beginning to look much more fertile for tobacco-control efforts nationwide. The 1998 Master Settlement Agreement between the tobacco industry and forty-six states was about to inject more than $200 billion into state coffers. The hope that some of this money would be used for prevention and treatment of addiction to cigarettes was stirring new thinking in many state health agencies. Other national organizations were also sponsoring major anti-tobacco programs, though not with a consistent focus on legislative change. Within the Robert Wood Johnson Foundation, the combination of compelling research, growing public support, and early successes in states like Alaska and Hawaii was creating momentum for a stronger policy agenda. Together, this mix of favorable conditions provided the burst of energy that set a midcourse correction in motion.

"As time went on and the social milieu changed around smoking, the momentum began to pick up to make these changes," Kaufman recalls. "States were in financial trouble, and they needed revenue they could get from cigarette taxes. Some of our [Foundation-sponsored] research was on public opinion, and it was showing widespread support for this source of revenue, unlike other kinds of tax increases. We could demonstrate that the economic effects of clean-indoor-air laws weren't negative—they could actually be positive. Everything was gathering force around this one conclusion. States were ready for it. A lot of grantees were ready for it. Research and public opinion were behind it. So we had our answer: Focus only on policy change."

The revised program would train and support coalitions in advocating for the two policy measures shown to be most effective in reducing smoking by young people: higher cigarette taxes and clean-indoor-air laws. And it would try to do so in all fifty states. (It also supported a third measure—coverage of smoking-cessation efforts—though this was a lower priority.)

The Foundation's trustees approved a reengineered version of SmokeLess States—$52 million over three years—in July 2000. (The program would eventually become one of the Foundation's biggest ever, totaling nearly $100 million over its ten-year life span.)

This refocusing and expansion would be an operational challenge in more than the usual ways. Changing public policy is not just a public-education task; it also calls for translating informed public opinion into successful legislation. Yet a direct appeal to lawmakers to enact specific laws (otherwise known as lobbying) is something that by law the Foundation could not support with its resources.

The prohibition on the use of Foundation funds for lobbying meant that the only way for coalitions to succeed in the legislative arena would be for them to raise other dollars that were not similarly restricted. They had been required to raise such matching money from the beginning, but in the next round the matching requirement would increase. The focus on policy change, in other words, would not only impose a new and tighter set of priorities on grantees, and require more of them to master the complex skills of effective advocacy, but would also require them to raise more money from additional sources.

Foundation grants could pay for the basic arsenal of effective advocacy: research, public education, advertising, media relations, the testimony of expert witnesses. The one thing it could not pay for was the actual firing of the weapons—that is, any use of these various assets to promote a particular bill or encourage others to promote it. That critical element of the campaign would have to be funded with outside support, particularly membership dues from partner organizations such as the American Cancer Institute and the American Heart Association. "We worked very, very hard before the next call for proposals to help people understand how important the matching funds were, and ways they could think about raising them," according to Michelle Larkin, one of the program officers overseeing the program and the current head of the Foundation's public health team.

As the program officers drafted the new call for proposals, they set out to help grantees brace for the changes. "We sent experts to states [that weren't in the program previously] to help them form coalitions," Larkin says. "We had conference calls with different organizations to help them sort out their turf issues. This wasn't just a call for proposals to see what we got; it was a ton of work to get people to truly understand—at the national level and among all of our partner organizations—what we were trying to achieve and how we would have to work together to do that."

The narrower focus, the newly precise performance goals, and a nationwide expansion of the program would also impose a major new workload on what was then a relatively small national program office, based at the American Medical Association. In 2000, Kaufman recruited Donna Grande, a leader of the Arizona coalition and former head of the National Cancer Institute's $128 million tobacco-control initiative, to become the deputy director of the program. Grande's management savvy and her experience in advocacy seemed a valuable complement to the organizational and team-building skills of the program's director, Thomas Houston. Within a year, when the new round of funding was announced, the office expanded its staff and began deploying people in field offices around the country. Grande became co-director with Houston, yet another sign of the importance of the implementation challenges the expansion was imposing.

Thanks partly to the advance work in preparing grantees for change, and partly to the improved political environment nationally, the new, expanded program quickly showed signs of meeting its performance goals. "There was a huge, dramatic change in a short amount of time," Grande says. The escalation in Foundation support, the surge in matching grants for direct support of legislation, and the growing list of states and localities with antismoking laws all combined to shift the movement into high gear. "A lot of advances, a lot of good things were visibly happening. But did it come easy and natural? No."

In fact, the demanding performance measurements— numerical targets for how much tobacco taxes would rise and how many clean-indoor-air laws would be passed, among other things—struck many people as unrealistic when the first new call for proposals was circulated. Karen Gerlach, a former Foundation senior program officer who, with Larkin, oversaw the SmokeLess States program, recalls, "When we first presented them, people said 'You'll never do that.' But we met the tax objective a year early. The number of states with comprehensive clean-indoor-air laws at the time wasn't even half a dozen. Now it's more than twenty. Well over half of the US population is protected by comprehensive clean-indoor-air laws." Although the Foundation was far from the only agent behind this change, it had seized the initiative at an opportune moment, adding powerful fuel to a newly smoldering fire.

Just as important, the Foundation was building a national argument, a rationale for action that helped galvanize further support and build momentum. From the time the goals were set, Gerlach says, "we translated them into lives saved: Increase the tax by x, and that will drive [tobacco] use rates down by y, which means that z people won't die of smoking-related disease."

But those accomplishments came with a sharply higher price tag, and with a significant increase in workload for both the Foundation and many of its grantees. The key to sustaining the energy behind all the additional work and expenditure, Gerlach says, was constant communication among the Foundation, the national program office at the American Medical Association, and the grantees—not only at the time of grantmaking but throughout the implementation as well. "We did an ungodly number of site visits," she says. "Way more after the change than before. Not just the national program office—the Foundation staff went, too. The advisory committee went. It wasn't just left up to the national program office to tell us how a coalition was doing."

In all of this, she concludes, "Communication is the big lesson. Deciding to make a change was easy. Figuring out how the change would work was harder. But bringing everyone into the change, making sure everyone understood it, bought into it, knew how they were going to fulfill their obligations—that was the really hard part. And without it, none of the rest would have mattered."

—∿— Design Flaws: Fixing a Strategy that Doesn't Match Reality

When the federal welfare reform act was passed, in 1996, its defenders argued that even though public assistance would now be restricted, many other safety-net programs would be available to soften the blow. Most former recipients would still be eligible for health benefits from Medicaid and the State Children's Health Insurance Program, known as SCHIP; for nutrition programs like food stamps; and for income support through the earned income tax credit, among other subsidies. Yet by the end of the decade, studies were beginning to show that as many as two-thirds of people leaving welfare were not receiving support from these other programs for which they were eligible. In the areas of health and nutrition, subjects of particular concern to the Robert Wood Johnson Foundation, the consequences for families and children seemed likely to be severe and long-lasting.

Beginning in 2000, the Foundation's Covering Kids program* set out to close this gap by enrolling eligible children in Medicaid and SCHIP. A related program, called Supporting Families After Welfare Reform, aimed squarely at the administrative nuts and bolts of the eligibility process: the procedural and technical roadblocks that prevent families from receiving benefits. Michael Rothman, who had been a manager in state government before joining the Foundation staff as a senior program officer, took a keen interest in the operational details of the eligibility maze.

"I knew that the way things were executed was as important as what the nominal rules or policies were," he says. "There could be ways you could implement the same rules in two counties or states that would have a big effect on how you miss people who should be enrolled, or enroll people who shouldn't be. So our strategy was to get straight into the day-to-day management

---

* In 2001, the program was expanded and renamed Covering Kids & Families.

and implementation issues with a technical assistance program for states and counties."

The program he designed started with a diagnostic phase, in which administrators from seven states and counties gathered to examine the means by which people became eligible for Medicaid and how their eligibility determinations were handled. In this phase, management consultants guided grantees (most of which were state or county health and social services agencies) through a painstaking exercise aimed at mapping their administrative procedures, scrutinizing administrative data, identifying flaws and obstacles in the eligibility process, and highlighting the ones that could readily be changed. Afterward, policy consultants would help grantees' staff members devise solutions to be implemented in the program's final stage. The Southern Institute on Children and Families, which served as the national program office for the Covering Kids and later the Covering Kids & Families initiatives, also took responsibility for Supporting Families.

Unfortunately, the diagnostic exercise proved to be more burdensome than useful. The mapping-and-analysis regimen, a new approach that the consultants were pilot testing in this program, dragged on for months, often perplexing the state and county officials taking part in it. Rothman shared their frustration: "If you're itching for change and results, as I tend to be, this kind of thing can be a little much. We'd been planning for six months, and there was not one more person enrolled in Medicaid or SCHIP. And I was concerned that we were making grantees spend a lot of their time analyzing their navel."

Worse, the data on which the navel gazing was based turned out to be nearly meaningless. Carolyn Needleman, then a professor at Bryn Mawr College and the program's evaluator, saw grantees devoting hundreds of person hours to eking data out of archaic, jury-rigged government databases. "It came as a big surprise to everyone that state computer systems aren't everything we think they are," she says. Consultants and the national program office staff members "thought it would just be a matter of going to the computer and pulling data according to a standard template and then working with the policy consultants to design an intervention. There was no recognition that states are working with antiquated equipment, where the whole system is built on all kinds of patches and workarounds."

The final blow to the program's design came in the economic avalanche of the 2001 recession, whose consequences delivered a body blow to state budgets in the 2002 fiscal year—just when Supporting Families' diagnostic and planning phase was supposed to wrap up. By the end of 2001, after three quarters of market decline, steep job losses, and plummeting tax revenue, it was all but unimaginable that state governments would cooperate with any effort to enlarge their already swelling safety net programs.

But the adverse effects of a harsh economy—largely the result of the terrorist attacks of September 11—were an external surprise, largely unforeseeable, not a defect of the underlying model. The more basic problem with the Supporting Families strategy, as Lavizzo-Mourey summed it up later, was that "there was a theory of how we could use data to make the [eligibility] system work better, and that theory was fundamentally flawed." By the beginning of 2002, Rothman had concluded that the program would have to change in essential ways.

At that point, it was also time for him to present to his Foundation colleagues the results of the program's opening phase, including a cautionary first-year report from the evaluators. It would not have been unusual for such a presentation to remain upbeat and noncommittal—the program was still new, a few bugs were only to be expected, and the diagnostic tool was being refined. Instead, he chose to deliver the news unvarnished: Some of the program's assumptions didn't match reality, it needed a new approach, and the national economy was making matters much tougher. "It was unusual to have that kind of conversation," Rothman admits, noting that senior Foundation officials, confronted with unexpected bad news, can sometimes panic, inferring that things might be even worse than they seem.

Luckily, he was prepared with a credible midcourse correction. Through his work on a separate Foundation program, aimed at promoting quality improvement in hospital care, Rothman had observed a promising technique for helping professionals work in teams to quickly identify problems, design better practices, and implement them immediately. He reasoned that this same technique, known as the Breakthrough Series and developed by the Boston-based Institute for Healthcare Improvement (IHI), could likewise help state and county administrators improve their eligibility processes quickly and concretely. It would surely be a more reliable way of identifying systemic problems and devising solutions than the fruitless yearlong scrutiny of administrative data had been.

By unveiling the Breakthrough Series model at the meeting with his colleagues, Rothman quickly turned a discussion about disappointment into one about fresh ideas and opportunity. He presented the new approach as a timely pivot, early in an evolving program, to capitalize on the first year's lessons and to preserve the grantees' enthusiasm and momentum. His colleagues, Rothman thinks, "may have seen some candor and flexibility and alacrity in that. They probably saw it as good that we were being open." Any sense of alarm quickly faded, and the program went forward with broad support.

The Breakthrough Series focuses expressly on "small tests of change"—hypothetical quality improvements, even on a tiny scale, that can be put in place immediately, judged quickly, and scaled up if they work. The process entails a brief period of learning and discussion on a given area of improvement, followed by repeated, rapid cycles known as PDSA, for "plan, do, study, act." Participants start by planning improvements that seem to make sense and positing some way of measuring whether they will work. The plans are implemented on a small scale and quickly evaluated (those are the "do" and "study" phases). Then, in the final "act" stage, participants either correct mistakes or, if the tests worked, apply the corrections more broadly.

In April 2002, staff from the Southern Institute attended IHI's Breakthrough Series College, where they learned to conduct Breakthrough Series sessions for Supporting Families grantees. For roughly the next two years, they rebuilt the program around the PDSA cycles, with increasingly visible, if mostly small, effects. These included some improvements in eligibility rules, smoother work flows with less duplication in processing and decision making, and improved communication among agency staff.

As Carolyn Needleman put it, the small tests of change "weren't going to expand enrollment significantly—nobody made headway with that in such a bad economic environment. But they probably made families' experience with the eligibility process better. They probably helped avoid families getting improperly dropped from the rolls; and they improved the quality of service in agencies short of staff." The program ended in 2004—too soon for most of the Breakthrough results to be scaled up or turned into more thoroughgoing change.

Strangely, the program never completely abandoned its unpromising quest for administrative data. National program office staff members continued to press participating agencies for monthly data submissions, even though most grantees considered the exercise pointless. As Needleman notes, "One lesson is that any midcourse correction may well carry over baggage from the original model—practices and procedures that are inconsistent with the new approach, or at least aren't helpful, but are hard to break." In this case, long after the strategy of Supporting Families had veered away from dissecting reams of computer output, the grant requirements continued to call for regular data dumps, month after month, apparently in the hope that someday the numbers might reveal something. Changing strategy, in other words, may be difficult, but changing the way of doing business is harder. It can be a mistake to assume that the first will automatically lead to the second.

More generally, participants in Supporting Families believe that the fundamental lesson of this course correction was the need for program designers to pay close attention to the day-to-day activity taking place under a grant, listen to the assessments of those implementing a program, and be alert to problems that can be remedied before they drag on too long.

A second lesson, emphasized by both Rothman and Needleman, is that programs are likely to be stronger if they build the possibility of course corrections into their basic model, so that the people managing them are ready to learn and adjust strategy as circumstances evolve, rather than treating any change as a sign of trouble. "It's not necessarily a flaw if a program needs to change course," Needleman concludes. "Especially if a program is aimed at public policy change. In that case, the point is to seize policy opportunities, and those come and go. So strategies have to adapt. If it comes to be expected that you're going to have evolving strategies, if the program is designed with enough flexibility so that it naturally shifts course when circumstances change, that could be a better way to approach public policy initiatives." As Michael Rothman found in candidly sharing with his colleagues his plans to reshape Supporting Families, the availability of a prompt, credible course correction can actually build confidence in a faltering program—provided that the correction is timely, well thought out, and persuasive.

—ᴧᴧ— Failure to Execute: Trying to Fix a Faltering Strategy by Changing the Implementation

For the sake of discussion, imagine a multiyear program to improve health outcomes for chronically homeless people—call it Safe Harbor. Let's say the program's strategy involved forming coalitions of health, housing, substance abuse, and social service agencies in states and large metropolitan areas. The coalitions were expected to propose, advocate for, and implement system changes that would integrate health care, addiction treatment, and mental health services for homeless adults and families. (This is an imaginary program that combines real events from Foundation initiatives in other fields. None of these programs had anything to do with homelessness. Any resemblance to actual organizations or work in the field of homelessness is purely accidental.)**

For the national program office, the Foundation picked a well-known mental health agency where a senior executive, a widely respected psychiatrist, would serve as program director. Her credentials included years of experience treating mentally ill homeless people and directing clinical programs in communities with high rates of homelessness. Yet the choice was not unanimous among program staff at the Foundation. Some officers expressed concern that the staff at the mental health agency was not sufficiently experienced in the fiscal and political challenges of trying to combine such disparate public systems.

"To us, the biggest challenge [for the national director] was not going to be the specific content expertise," said one senior program officer, referring to expertise in particular kinds of service delivery. "That's widely available. To us, the challenge was in mobilizing the various sectors of a community to work together on a common problem. We needed people with experience in political science and political organization. But there was a difference of opinion [within the Foundation] on the skill set needed." Despite these objections, senior officers ratified the selection, and the trustees authorized Safe Harbor for an initial four-year phase, combining up to two years of organizing and planning with two to three years of implementation.

Throughout the early organization and planning stage, most coalitions' work was too preliminary to judge its effectiveness, though clearly there was considerable ferment in many communities. In fact, the issue of homelessness and health was becoming

---

** The reason for using a fictional program is primarily to avoid reigniting old conflicts and embarrassing the individuals involved. Throughout this description, every quote and event described is real, but they have been woven together from different stories and periods of time, and occasional words have been changed to disguise the specific programs and people under discussion.

a subject of national concern in these years. Many in the Foundation believed they were riding, or perhaps leading, a national wave of activity in the field. Perhaps as a result, there was a tendency to view the early years of the program as promising—an exertion of national leadership on an important issue—even though the actual coalitions were often slow to form, troubled by simmering turf issues, and inconsistent in their ability to draw real decision makers to meetings.

Furthermore, Foundation assets were growing at this time, and more resources encouraged even more ambitious ideas. "I pushed to bring more sites on, even though I'm not sure there was any evidence it was going to work," a top Foundation executive acknowledges. "It was a very ambitious program, relative to the budget." After the planning and trial phases, the trustees approved a second four-year round of funding for full implementation.

By this stage, however, program officers and evaluators were beginning to report more and more disquieting news from the field. Coalitions that supposedly had rallied around clear plans and strategies actually seemed, on close observation, to be simply endorsing or expanding projects that members had been operating for years. In other cases, groups seemed to have been taken over by a few powerful members pushing their own agendas, with little participation from the rest of the group.

"There was a sense of entitlement at the national program office and among the staff of some of the larger grantees in the field, and they didn't seem to be worrying much about quality," another program officer observed. "We would go to [local] meetings where people said, 'We're the coalition.' But then members would start showing up one by one and introducing themselves to the other people in the room. This was years after they were first funded, and they didn't all even know one another! How were they supposed to be collaborating? This was way before e-mail was common."

Near the end of the second four-year funding authorization, evaluators not only confirmed what the program officers were observing on site visits but also added discouraging data of their own, showing that the coalitions' work was often ensnared in the conflicting missions and priorities of their member organizations, resulting in little visible change in service delivery or coordination. Discouragement with Safe Harbor was by now so acute that some senior executives at the Foundation were ready to reduce the program severely or even pull the plug at the end of the second round, by which time almost a decade would have passed. Yet the Foundation staff members leading the effort reminded their colleagues that the leadership of the national program office had never been their preferred choice to implement the model. Just as they had warned from the beginning, the leaders of the national program office had proven more skilled as clinicians and scholars than as agents of political change. They had focused too much on recruiting broad coalitions and minimizing dissent and disaffection. They had been reluctant to pressure the coalitions into making difficult choices, shouldering the burdens of an action campaign, and achieving concrete results.

"We didn't want to declare it a failure when we hadn't even given it the chance of having the right leadership," one senior program officer at the Robert Wood Johnson Foundation said. "I felt strongly that you can't declare something unworkable unless you've given it a chance to work—which you haven't done if you've given it to the wrong person." In the end, that argument carried the day, despite some skepticism from a few members of the Foundation's management. Shortly thereafter, a top-level delegation was dispatched to convey the news to the national program director that someone else would soon be taking the helm.

"That was a very painful conversation," a Foundation official recalls. "But we owed it to her to be straight with her, not to play games. That would have been literally adding insult to injury. The fact that we went in person, and that one member of the team had worked with her for years and had tremendous interpersonal skills—that helped some. It was one more step to soften the blow without beating around the bush."

Softened or not, the blow was felt throughout the national program office and around the field, including among many project managers who were personally fond of the director. It took considerable time to heal those hard feelings, and some never healed at all. "As the transition took place," a Foundation program officer observes, the new director "was a little tougher on the sites. Some of them looked back fondly on the good old days with [the first director], who would hold their hand and tell them how wonderful they were." The new program director, by contrast, "would always say, 'Where's the data?' Which is what we had always wanted to ask."

Besides the new national program director, other aspects of the program were overhauled as well. The national program office was given a more visible, guiding role in the field, shepherding the coalitions (and prodding them, where necessary) from planning toward action. The program's national advisory committee was restructured to include more members with experience in organizing system-change movements—experience that would in turn be made available to the national program office and to the coalitions in the field. In the next round of grants, the call for proposals made much clearer the kinds of accomplishments that grantees would be expected to show and the kinds of help they would receive from the national program office in reaching those goals. Funding, thenceforward, depended on evidence that public opinion was becoming more strongly supportive, that new policies were advancing or enacted, and that more homeless people were receiving better coordinated, efficient, and effective care.

By this time, however, it seems that the patterns were largely set in many of the participating coalitions. The new national program director had the unenviable job of trying to reverse long-standing habits at many sites, though by then, a few coalitions did have a basis of real accomplishment to build on. In any case, by the time the program ended, several years later, opinions on its success were mixed.

(In reality, the programs from which this composite story was made had varying degrees of success with their midterm tactical shifts. One case ended markedly better than it began; others continued to drift, though to some eyes they were much more effective than they would have been had the course of implementation not been changed. "We can all speculate about 'what if,' says an observer of two of these cases. "But the truth is, we have no evidence to say what would have happened had the choices been different.")

The two main lessons of these experiences, several participants seem to agree, are, first, that it's essential to think through implementation issues at the time the program is being designed, and to be sure the designated leaders have the right skills from the beginning. Second, program staff members should look closely and continually at how implementation is proceeding at the front lines. Simply reading year-end reports or observing a program too casually from afar could deprive the Foundation of the ability to correct problems before it's too late. As a participant in one of these cases put it, "Someone who's right [as a program leader] at the very beginning, when the challenge is mainly formative and capacity-building, may be completely wrong later on, when things have to be driven by hard objectives."

—w— Lessons and Principles

In a 2007 report to The James Irvine Foundation on a program that had undergone a midcourse correction, the consultant Gary Walker observed that "early implementation problems . . . are not unusual in large-scale initiatives."[1]

No formula exists to resolve the hard questions: Should anything be done? By whom? When? Answers are particular to the initiative. It is tempting to assert that arriving at the answers is a simple matter of continuous staff diligence. When implementation issues arise, an organization's best bet is to have enlisted enough capable, experienced staff and to have incorporated a regular executive and board review.

Yet like the programs profiled here, the Irvine initiative Walker was studying already "had all of these elements: smart, capable staff and regular executive and board reviews." The problem wasn't care and intelligence, he concluded, but something more basic to the culture of large-scale philanthropy: "The forces, structure, and incentives of the philanthropic world are geared toward staying the course—or expanding the course. The call for more time, resources, and technical assistance is not an unusual large-foundation response to an initiative's early or midcourse problems."[2]

Nearly all the programs examined here succumbed to these same temptations for a time. Except for Supporting Families, the others were renewed and enlarged before they were revamped. All of them either discounted or overlooked early warning signs that expectations were not matching reality. Yet all the programs, including those blended into the composite case, eventually confronted reality and rethought some of their earliest, most basic decisions.

Five factors seem to be critical to bringing about that kind of honest reckoning. Some of them, had they been considered earlier in the program's life cycle, might have made for a more timely, efficient, and maybe effective program than what eventually unfolded. But all of them proved valuable eventually. And as Walker pointed out, that is not common in large-scale philanthropy. The following are, in distilled form, five key recommendations that participants in these cases offer for spotting problems earlier, dealing with them effectively, and making sure, as a program observer in our composite case put it, that "you don't declare something unworkable unless you've given it a chance to work."

> 1. *Be prepared to change a program's direction—even in relatively early stages—if performance is not meeting expectations.* As the evaluator Carolyn Needleman put it, "It's not necessarily a flaw if a program needs

to change course." Some program designs confront known risks that can be closely monitored from the beginning. Deliberate attention to these risks and a willingness to respond with a timely change of course can be the best way to stave off more consequential problems later. Yet even when risks can't be fully assessed up front, programs need a series of reassessment points, at which strategic choices are reopened and new approaches considered if performance is not meeting expectations. When these periodic reassessments are part of the original design, there is more of a chance that course corrections will be seen, in Michael Rothman's words, as "candor and flexibility and alacrity," rather than as a scramble to save face.

2. *Think early about the management skills that will be needed to execute a program effectively—especially if unforeseen problems arise and major changes have to be made down the road.* The choice of a national program director is often made on the basis of his or her vision, inventiveness, and outstanding performance on other programs. Yet in any new program, the odds are good that the gritty, tactical decisions in a long implementation will demand agility in management and communication even more than strategic vision, and that any given implementation process will raise problems unknown in other contexts. Picking implementers for their tactical dexterity as well as their substantive insight is one way to be sure that problems of execution are spotted early, on the front lines, and corrected deftly, without needless disruption to the program.

3. *Once a program is launched, stay in close contact with frontline actors and listen carefully to their impressions—don't wait for evaluation reports to learn what those on the front lines know all along.* Undoubtedly the most exciting work in philanthropy

is creating new initiatives, and many program officers candidly acknowledge that most of their creative energy goes into designing the next major program. Monitoring existing programs is time-consuming and operationally difficult (the presence of funders on a site can be unsettling to staff members, whose behavior can change markedly when grant makers appear at the door). Yet the information path from front lines to central headquarters can be long, tortuous, and full of distorting noise. There is no substitute, several grant makers and observers concluded, for a regular firsthand look at what's happening and candid discussions with the people who make it happen.

4. *Ensure that programs have frequent injections of independent judgment—from interim performance assessments, ongoing data analysis, and grantee feedback—to inform midcourse reviews.* The earlier and more often a program hears from evaluators, the more useful the evaluation is likely to be. Also, the jolt of an unexpected outside observation—positive or negative—can be an effective way of overcoming the inertia that sets in when programs last for many years and rely on the same dedicated team of people who are deeply invested in its basic assumptions and methods. Evaluation is critical, but as the Foundation's Michelle Larkin observes, "Sometimes on-the-ground intelligence from grantees and key stakeholders is more timely and relevant in assessing how a program is doing."

5. *Cultivate candor and flexibility in all foundation programs, encouraging frequent discussions of alternative courses of action and rewarding astute course corrections when they're needed.* Several program officers in our sample cases expressed a common concern in philanthropy: that colleagues, senior officers, and

trustees sometimes draw harsh conclusions from any admission that programs aren't progressing as planned, and that program officers' reputations can therefore suffer as a consequence. Most managers and trustees would probably recoil at such a perception, and work hard to rebut it. But it is widely held in the foundation world. It's true that foundations usually do a good job of cultivating independent, creative thought when programs are first being conceived—when the rail lines are being planned and laid, when engines and cars are being designed and purchased. The harder, but equally crucial, challenge is to create the same atmosphere of critical thinking, versatility, and honesty when the time comes to pull up the tracks and aim the engines in a new direction.

One way to make that happen, according to the Robert Wood Johnson Foundation president and CEO, Risa Lavizzo-Mourey, is to focus staff attention on performance and impact throughout the life of a program, not just as it nears its conclusion. "Gauging progress and impact regularly forces you to re-examine your theory of change, and at least ask the question whether you are on the trajectory that you should be on, given your theory," she says. "And if you're not, why not, given the environment? You need a system that regularly calls for assessing progress, even when it's too soon to see impact. And that system has to be open, encouraging, and routine, so staff will see it as a part of the creative process, not as a report card where they are going to pass or fail."

Notes

1. Walker, G. *Midcourse Corrections to a Major Initiative: A Report on the James Irvine Foundation's CORAL Initiative*. The James Irvine Foundation, May 2007.
2. Ibid.

CHAPTER 3

The National Health Care Purchasing Institute: A Case Study

Michael H. Brown

"Experience is the name everyone gives to their mistakes," wrote the Irish playwright Oscar Wilde.[1] This is the story of a $7.7 million experience named the National Health Care Purchasing Institute—a Robert Wood Johnson Foundation program that ended unhappily for just about everyone: the Foundation, the program staff, and the constituency the program was to help.

Authorized by the Foundation's board in 1999, the program trained health care purchasing executives to use their buying power to improve the quality and cost-effectiveness of health care. That, at least, was the purpose. In 2002, after a little more than three of the program's intended five years, the Robert Wood Johnson Foundation decided to close the Purchasing Institute and shift the remaining funds to a different purchasing reform effort. For the Foundation, it was a rare occasion of terminating a program early.

—ᴍ— Value-Based Purchasing of Health Care

Discontent with the quality and the cost of American health care was widespread in corporate America in the 1990s. Simply put, executives felt that their companies and employees were not getting their money's worth for the millions spent on health care. The Institute of Medicine's 1999 report, *To Err Is Human,* grabbed headlines with the estimate that as many as 98,000 hospital patients were dying each year from preventable medical errors. But the statistic merely echoed a refrain previously heard in boardrooms and executive suites: the American health care system was unreliable and inefficient.

Indeed, instead of rewarding quality care, the system often penalized it, especially for the treatment of chronic conditions. For example, a medical practice that carefully tracked its diabetic patients was unlikely to be reimbursed for the extra effort. A hospital that helped congestive heart patients manage their illness on an outpatient basis ran the risk of reducing admissions and profitability. The problem was by no means confined to private businesses. Critics contended that the Medicare payment system—reimbursing providers for procedures and services— encouraged treatment without regard for quality.

Some businesses—mainly large corporations—decided to do more than just complain. Instead of continuing to funnel checks to health plans and providers with no questions asked, they began using their economic clout to influence the effectiveness of the coverage they subsidized for their workers, retirees, and dependents. This activist approach came to be known as *value-based purchasing.* Negotiating price discounts is, of course, as old as business itself. The goal of value-based purchasing, however, is to improve the quality of health care, not just the cost—in short, to get greater value for the health care dollar.

There are different strategies for doing that. One approach is to reward providers for improving their care processes and outcomes—called pay for performance. The idea is to give health care organizations a financial stake in meeting guidelines shown to result in improved patient health status, and a number of companies tried it. Acting alone or through purchasing coalitions, they identified best clinical practices, set performance measures, and paid bonuses to health care organizations that met performance targets. Another approach is to adjust the premium share paid by employees to encourage their migration from low-performing plans to high-performing ones.

Although simple in concept, pay for performance and other value-based purchasing practices are not necessarily easy to implement. Determining what performance standards to apply and collecting the relevant data from providers can be a significant undertaking—both technically and financially. Another challenge is determining a valid relationship between incentives and improvement: Can money make a difference, and if so, how much does it take? While some corporations had the financial wherewithal and the motivation to tackle these tasks, purchasing reform remained beyond the reach of much of the private sector. Progress was even slower in government agencies, where funding limitations and legal requirements restricted purchasing practices.

—ɯ— Genesis of the National Health Care Purchasing Institute

It all started with Lynn Etheredge, a Washington consultant specializing in health care issues. Having held positions in the federal Office of Management and Budget during four administrations, he knew the ins and outs of Medicare and its need for modernization—including purchasing practices.

Etheredge wanted the Centers for Medicare & Medicaid Services (CMS)—then named the Health Care Financing Administration—to adopt the tactics of leading private-sector payers and use purchasing tools as part of the strategy for controlling costs and improving quality and service. However, he saw the culture of CMS as a major barrier to purchasing reform.

Many CMS employees, he said in an interview, spent their entire careers in the agency and had little or no exposure to private-sector purchasers. While well versed in writing regulations, most lacked experience in negotiating and related skills common to the competitive marketplace, he said.

Etheredge wanted to change that, and he had an idea for how: Train public-sector purchasers in the innovative purchasing practices of the private sector. Lacking an organization of his own that could run a training program, Etheredge took his idea to a long-time friend, W. David Helms, the founder and head of a Washington policy research and education organization then called the Alpha Center, which later became AcademyHealth. Helms had experience both in training public-sector officials and as a Robert Wood Johnson Foundation grantee, including management of the Foundation's long-running programs, State Coverage Initiatives and Changes in Health Care Financing and Organization.

Helms liked Etheredge's idea, and the two agreed to join forces to make it a reality. There was, however, a difference in the focus of the two men. Etheredge was interested in training that emphasized the techniques and practicalities of purchasing, and Helms was interested in combining substantive knowledge about purchasing with more generic leadership training. He saw an inequity between the leadership development opportunities available to top-level executives in the private sector and their counterparts in the public sector, and he thought the proposed program could help close that gap.

Etheredge and Helms took their idea to top CMS officials, including Bruce Vladeck, then head of the agency, and got an enthusiastic response. Helms recalls Vladeck saying that CMS didn't need another academic paper on purchasing but rather concrete assistance on how to apply private sector purchasing approaches within the public sector, with all of its rules and regulations regarding contracting. The two also contacted Nancy Barrand, a senior program officer at the Foundation at the time and currently the special adviser for program development, about getting a planning grant to flesh out the concept. Barrand arranged for the two to meet with the Foundation's executive vice president, Lewis Sandy, who agreed to provide planning money. In April 1997, Helms' organization, the Alpha Center, formally requested a grant to plan what the proposal called the National Leadership Purchasing Institute for Public Purchasing of Health Care. Six months later, the Foundation awarded a $364,000 planning grant.

—ᴡᴡ— The Robert Wood Johnson Foundation Context

Traditionally, purchasing and related business aspects of the health care delivery system have not been major grant making areas for the Robert Wood Johnson Foundation. However, increasing the value of health care dollars—especially those spent on the elderly, the poor, and other vulnerable populations—advances the heart of the Foundation's overall mission: to improve the health and health care of Americans. Thus, while something of an outlier in the Robert Wood Johnson Foundation's portfolio, a program to strengthen value-based purchasing tactics was by no means beyond the Foundation's spectrum of interests.

Indeed, the Foundation had previously invested in several efforts that touched directly on purchasing practices. For example, the Health Insurance Reform Project—a Foundation-supported initiative at George Washington University between 1995 and 2005—explored potential Medicare reforms dealing with the purchase and delivery of care for the chronically ill.[2] Over the years, the Foundation had also supported initiatives to contain health care costs—an issue obviously related to purchasing.

The Foundation's focus on value-based purchasing increased in 1998 with the addition of Michael Rothman to the program staff. Rothman previously worked for the state of Colorado on health programs, including Medicaid purchasing initiatives. The

Foundation hired him with the expectation that he would bring his purchasing expertise to bear on the Foundation's programming. Rothman was particularly interested in spurring quality improvement through pay for performance. "The reality is, we can't expect most providers to make major investments in learning how to improve quality and in hiring staff and making systemic changes if they are going to lose money doing it," he said in an interview published in the Foundation newsletter *Advances*.

—⚋— The Planning Process

As indicated by the name in the planning grant proposal—the National Leadership Purchasing Institute for Public Purchasing of Health Care—the objective of the program envisioned by Etheredge and Helms was to help government agencies and employees. The Foundation staff's written justification for the planning grant echoed that objective: "This project represents a special opportunity for the Foundation to build and improve the capacity of the public sector as a major purchaser of health care in order to improve quality of care as well as to contain costs."

Although Etheredge's emphasis was on Medicare, the training program would not be limited to Medicare. The target audience, according to the planning proposal, would be the staff of CMS, state Medicaid and State Children's Health Insurance Program (SCHIP) agencies, federal and state employee systems, and other public purchasers such as school districts, cities, and counties. The private sector would be involved as trainer but not trainee. Leading corporate purchasers would be on hand to provide expertise and offer networking opportunities to the public-sector participants.

In addition to Helms and Etheredge, the planning team included Susan O'Loughlin Ward, an independent consultant who previously had served as deputy administrator of the Washington State Health Care Authority, and Jack Ebeler, a former Clinton administration health official then working as a consultant to the Alpha Center. (Shortly thereafter, Ebeler joined the

Robert Wood Johnson Foundation as a senior vice president.) Barrand oversaw the planning for the Foundation, and an advisory committee of CMS executives, state Medicaid directors, and private-sector purchasers helped guide the effort. The planning team conducted meetings and telephone interviews with stakeholders to learn the challenges facing health care purchasers and the resources already available.

A major focus of the planning process was the development of a prototype training course. In a later interview, Barrand recalled that she and Helms differed somewhat on the proposed content for the course. She wanted the curriculum to emphasize hands-on problem solving, she said, while Helms was interested in attracting high-level officials and executives whose support for more detailed purchasing approaches would be required. Helms believed that this would require a combination of leadership-oriented content using case studies and technical content related to purchasing.

In the end, the course consisted of presentations and panel discussions on both leadership and purchasing practices. Helms' organization, the Alpha Center, pilot-tested the prototype in Winston-Salem, North Carolina, in November 1998. Fifty people from twenty public and private organizations attended the three-day course.

Reaction at CMS to the course was favorable. Nancy-Ann DeParle, CMS administrator at the time and a member of the Foundation's board of trustees between 2002 and 2009, when she resigned to accept a position as the director of the White House Office for Health Reform, wrote Helms that while she herself did not attend, "Our senior leadership has been abuzz ever since returning, and the experience was a real shot in the arm for the whole agency. I hope we can keep it going."

An Expanded Focus

In January 1999, the planning committee met to consider feedback from course attendees and arrive at a final program design.

The next month, the Alpha Center submitted a proposal to the Robert Wood Johnson Foundation for funding to implement what was now to be called the National Health Care Purchasing Institute. Although the name was shortened, the targeted audience was significantly enlarged. Instead of just public-sector purchasers, the implementation grant proposal called for the program also to train executives from large private purchasers, such as those from Fortune 100 companies.

The decision to some extent pitted the program's originators against a newer set of actors. Etheredge and Helms continued to believe that the Purchasing Institute should focus on just the public sector. "I didn't think the Robert Wood Johnson Foundation needed to spend its money helping GE and GM do a better job on purchasing," Helms said in a later interview. Barrand agreed, but as the planning grant was coming to a close, she took maternity leave, and Rothman, her replacement, favored opening the training to corporate purchasers. Including company executives as trainees and not just trainers, he said, would facilitate the exchange of ideas and expertise between the private and public sectors as well as enlarge the Purchasing Institute's potential impact on the entire marketplace. (Barrand returned to the Foundation several months later, but Rothman continued as the Purchasing Institute's program officer for the remainder of its existence.)

Kevin "Kip" Piper, who joined the Alpha Center staff during the planning period, was another voice in favor of including private purchasers. Piper previously headed Wisconsin's Bureau of Health Care Financing, and had been selected by Helms to direct the new training program if and when the funding materialized. A third influential voice for adding private purchasers was Bruce Bradley, a top health care official at General Motors and a member of the planning committee. Bradley argued that the corporate world did not have all the answers, and that private and public purchasers should participate on an equal footing. Casting private-sector purchasers in a teaching role only would smack of arrogance, he said in an interview.

Ultimately, the view of Bradley, Rothman, and Piper won out over that of Barrand, Helms, and Etheredge. As explained in the Alpha Center's final report to the Robert Wood Johnson Foundation on the planning grant results, "it became clear that the best way to effect a strong public-private partnership and provide the leadership needed for health care purchasing would be to add private purchasers to the target audience."

Two More Planning Issues

Medicaid. The initial concept of Etheredge and Helms envisioned Medicaid among the public-sector programs that the Purchasing Institute would benefit. Barrand, however, believed that Medicaid, which is administered by the states, was sufficiently different from federally run Medicare that a separate training program for Medicaid purchasers was needed. She proposed creating a Medicaid purchasing institute at the Center for Health Care Strategies, a New Jersey-based nonprofit health policy organization. The Center was already running the Medicaid Managed Care Program—a Foundation initiative to increase the ability of state Medicaid agencies to participate in managed care. Barrand saw Medicaid purchasing as a logical part of that effort.

Stephen Somers, president and chief executive officer of the Center and a former Robert Wood Johnson Foundation associate vice president, concurred. Many state Medicaid agencies, he said in an interview, were far ahead of Medicare in the transition to managed care, and thus had a different perspective on purchasing issues and training needs. Another factor, according to Somers, was that state Medicaid personnel tend to view CMS as a regulator, and would have been uncomfortable participating with CMS officials in joint training.

Helms and Etheredge resisted splitting off Medicaid, but the planning committee went along with Barrand and Somers. The result was apparently a kind of compromise. While the Foundation's files are silent on this aspect, interviews indicate that the plan was for the Purchasing Institute at the Alpha

Center to train state Medicaid directors in big-picture purchasing concepts while Somers' organization worked with the full state Medicaid teams—the directors and their underlings—on the more technical aspects of value-based purchasing.

Technical Assistance. There was also the question of whether the Purchasing Institute should emphasize generic leadership skills (Helms' preference) or technical purchasing know-how (Etheredge's).

Barrand, Rothman, and Bradley favored a practical focus. Rothman recalled that it was Bradley who first identified the Breakthrough Series as a metaphor for the kind of comprehensive technical assistance that the Purchasing Institute should provide. The Breakthrough Series is a collaborative learning system that the Institute for Healthcare Improvement in Cambridge, Massachusetts, developed to help organizations make fundamental—breakthrough—improvements in the quality of their care. Participating teams from hospitals and other institutions attend periodic group sessions to learn about system change from experts. In between sessions, the teams implement improvement projects at their home facilities, with technical assistance provided through conference calls, online dialogue, and site visits.

That was the model that Rothman wanted the Purchasing Institute to follow, he said in an interview after the program closed. To what degree the message got through is unclear, however. The program planning documents do not mention the Breakthrough Series, nor did the Alpha Center's proposal to the Robert Wood Johnson Foundation for implementation funding. Instead, it outlined plans for an annual "executive course" conducted in two stages: an initial three-day session on strategic, senior management-level purchasing issues and strategies, followed six months later by a session to reinforce the earlier material. There was no mention of team projects in between.

A separate description of the planned new program written by Foundation staff members for the board of trustees reflected

Rothman's view of how the curriculum should be structured: After the initial three-day session—which was to be a "problem-solving oriented course"—each participating executive would pursue a project aimed at bringing change to his or her home organization; at the follow-up course, the participants would share information about their efforts. Rothman said he discussed the value of this three-part approach with Piper. However, in hindsight, the fact that the Alpha Center proposal included a more limited course format should have given him pause about the organization's commitment to the Breakthrough Series model, he said.

Along with the annual course, the Alpha Center's grant proposal envisioned the Purchasing Institute's conducting three to four "advanced purchasing workshops" each year on purchasing problems and skills. It would also help create leadership development programs at collaborating universities, with the curriculum aimed at health care purchasers.

In addition to offering face-to-face instruction, the proposal called for the new entity to publish five to six technical monographs a year and develop a number of tools—including a Web site, a newsletter, and a mentoring system—to encourage networking and information sharing among purchasers. The proposal defined the target audience as top officials of CMS, chiefs of state Medicaid agencies and their deputies, executives of large companies, purchasers for large federal and state employee systems, such the California Public Employees' Retirement System, and leaders of purchasing alliances and consortiums, such as the Pacific Business Group on Health.

—⌁— Implementation

In April 1999, the Robert Wood Johnson Foundation awarded the Alpha Center a $7,699,000 grant to organize the National Health Care Purchasing Institute and operate it for sixty months—from May 1, 1999, to April 30, 2004. Piper, the director, had a support staff that eventually grew to about half a dozen. Etheredge and

Susan O'Loughlin Ward, the planning team member, were senior consultants.

Etheredge's Departure

This team, however, did not last long. In September 1999—five months after the Purchasing Institute began—Etheredge withdrew, voicing strong dissatisfaction with the program's direction. Among his complaints was that it was paying insufficient attention to the needs of CMS. Within the Foundation, Etheredge's angry departure raised concerns. Suddenly, the Purchasing Institute was without the chief intellectual force behind its creation. "It was a difficult start," Barrand said.

In addition, Ward reduced her involvement in the program after giving birth to twins in July 1999. Thus, early in the implementation stage, most of the key players in the planning process moved on, one way or another.

The National Advisory Committee

As is customary with Robert Wood Johnson Foundation programs, the Alpha Center and the Foundation established a national advisory committee to help guide the Purchasing Institute. Bradley, the GM executive on the planning advisory committee, stayed on, but most of the members were new. The twenty-member panel included health care experts from government, industry, academia, and the nonprofit world.

The committee was a distinguished group, but it never had a designated chair, and Piper's office convened only two meetings—in June of 2000 and 2001. One member, David Lansky, then president of the Foundation for Accountability, said the 2001 meeting featured a briefing by the program staff and an interesting discussion. But there was no process for turning the discussion into program input, he said. He considered the meeting a poor use of the members' time. The committee, Bradley said, withered away.

Relationship of the Two Institutes

The Robert Wood Johnson Foundation gave the Center for Health Care Strategies funding to create what was initially called the State Medicaid/SCHIP Purchasing Institute and later the CHCS Purchasing Institute. It held its first training session for state Medicaid personnel in March 2000, the month after the Alpha Center's National Health Care Purchasing Institute held its initial course.

While the two purchasing institutes were to be complementary, that did not work out. One reason, according to Rothman, was that state Medicaid directors didn't have time to attend two different training courses, and they preferred to participate as a team with their staff rather than attend a separate course. Based on the feedback, Foundation staff members and the two institutes concluded that dividing up Medicaid was unworkable. As a result, in 2000 the National Health Care Purchasing Institute dropped state Medicaid agencies from its target audience.

The staffs of the two purchasing institutes did maintain contact, sending representatives to each other's training sessions and advisory committee meetings. Also, twice a year they met together with Foundation staff members to review progress. Nevertheless, the two institutes had different audiences and took different approaches to the training mission. As a result, there was little or no operational collaboration between the two, according to staff members of both.

Performance Measurement

The grant proposal laid out an ambitious plan to measure the Purchasing Institute's performance and impact. The Purchasing Institute was to track:

- Purchasing improvement among purchasing professionals, including changes in their knowledge and skills and in the number using value-based practices

■ Improvement in purchasing organizations, including the speed and ease with which organizations were
adapting to market changes and new technologies

The Purchasing Institute staff did conduct certain process
evaluations, such as tallying assessment forms filled out by course
participants, and also drafted an evaluation matrix that identified
goals and corresponding evaluation methods. However, the work
did not result in any meaningful measurement of the program's
impact on purchasing practices in the field.

A second, more concrete kind of evaluation also did not
materialize. While some "scholarships" were to be available, the
grant proposal foresaw a schedule of gradually increasing fees that
course participants would pay. The fees were to be a funding
source to help the Purchasing Institute become self-sufficient. In
addition, fees—or, more precisely, the degree to which individuals
and organizations were willing to pay them—also would have
helped gauge the program's usefulness.

In fact, course fees were never charged. Budget restrictions at
the attendees' home organizations would have made fees difficult
to implement, Piper said.

—∿— Results

Courses

The Purchasing Institute conducted three three-day courses
between 2000 and 2002. The Foundation's decision to close the
program scuttled plans for a fourth course in 2003. While called
courses, the sessions followed a conference format, with presentations and panel discussions. About fifty-five people—including
paid speakers—attended each year, representing a mixture of
public and private sector organizations.

There were no follow-up sessions, nor did attendees undertake projects in their home organizations. Corporate purchasers
did not have the time or the budget for additional commitments,

and getting the same people back together again would have been logistically difficult, according to Piper. Moreover, CMS's bureaucratic complexities would have defeated attempts to implement individual improvement projects at that agency.

In addition, the Purchasing Institute conducted nine workshops—each lasting one to two days and drawing about thirty-five to forty-five people—and held about half a dozen roundtable discussions, briefings, and other meetings. The idea of complementary university-based leadership programs, as outlined by the proposal, did not materialize because, Piper said, of the cost and scheduling difficulties of working with universities.

Communications

The staff commissioned and disseminated about twenty monographs and policy briefs written by consultants and academics on purchasing issues and strategies. A program Web site provided access to the reports and course agendas and links to other materials of potential interest to purchasers. By the program's third year, the site was averaging a little more than 300 visitors a day, the staff reported. Eight issues of the program newsletter, *Health Care Purchaser,* went to a mailing list of 1,800.

Non-Training Activities

With the Robert Wood Johnson Foundation's encouragement, the Purchasing Institute increasingly devoted resources to activities that went beyond training. For example, it provided funds and staff to support the formation of what became the Consumer-Purchaser Disclosure Project, a partnership focused on developing a system of publicly reported health care performance information.

Most notably, in the summer of 2001, the Purchasing Institute staff helped Rothman develop a new national program named Rewarding Results: Aligning Incentives with High-Quality

Health Care. This $7.5-million initiative, authorized by the Foundation's board of trustees in January 2002, supported demonstrations of pay-for-performance systems. Given Piper's involvement in planning the new program and its relevance to value-based purchasing, Rothman chose Piper to direct Rewarding Results in addition to the Purchasing Institute, and the Foundation made the Alpha Institute the national program office. Getting Rewarding Results under way—including overseeing the selection of seven demonstration sites—was a major, if not dominant, focus of the Purchasing Institute staff throughout 2002, its last year of operation.

—ᴧᴧ— Response

Response to the Purchasing Institute and its educational efforts was at best mixed according to interviews with participants and observers. For example, Helen Darling, president of the National Business Group on Health and a member of the planning advisory committee, said the reports disseminated by the program were well done but general in nature, more like policy reports put out by the Congressional Research Service than training documents that could provide concrete help to federal and state government purchasers.

Vincent Kerr, a physician who was director of health care management for the Ford Motor Company and later an executive of United Healthcare National Accounts, said the written materials ranged widely—from useless reiterations of what was already available to valuable tools. He found the training sessions helpful but wondered how many purchasers who attended actually changed practices as a result.

DeParle, the former CMS administrator and Foundation trustee, said that while she had high hopes for the Purchasing Institute, she found that a course she attended in 2000 lacked focus and substance. It had "a soft, touchy-feel to it," she said, making her wonder if this was a good use of CMS employees' time.

Robert Berenson, a top CMS official under President Clinton, echoed DeParle. The 1998 prototype and the 2000 courses were both good introductory meetings, Berenson said, but the program never progressed beyond that. "There was no meat," he said. "People started saying, 'I've got better things to do.'"

Not everyone was critical. Patricia Salber, a physician who was director of managed care health initiatives at General Motors and a speaker at a number of Purchasing Institute programs, said the attendees, whom she described as mainly midlevel executives, appeared to get a lot out of the sessions, and she herself found the Purchasing Institute reports helpful. Patricia MacTaggart, a former CMS official who worked with the Purchasing Institute staff, said the program played a beneficial role by bringing CMS and private-sector purchasers together to exchange views and expertise. But after two years, instead of more courses and white papers, what was needed was direct action to mobilize the purchasing field, she said.

Arnold Milstein, medical director of the Pacific Business Group on Health and chief physician for Mercer Health & Benefits, said the program worked well initially but then lost its "spark and excitement" and became stagnant. The program could have incubated enlightened purchasing practices by providing concrete technical assistance in the field, but it never did that, said Milstein, a member of the national advisory committee.

—ᴧᴧ— Closure

Dissatisfaction at the Robert Wood Johnson Foundation

Rothman wanted the curriculum to include multiple sessions interspersed with technical assistance and improvement projects. The Medicaid training program run by the Center for Health Care Strategies took that approach, he said, but the Alpha Center, which housed the Purchasing Institute, did not. Rothman saw that as significant. What he did not see also bothered him: evidence that the courses, workshops, reports, and other products were having an impact. The Purchasing Institute, he concluded, was failing to strengthen health care purchasing in either the public or private sector.

Rothman said he talked to Piper about the program's short-comings but, in hindsight, realized that he should have been more aggressive. Looking back, Rothman said, he saw that he also made another mistake: he never expressed his concerns to Helms.

An Alternative Emerges

In contrast to what he perceived to be the Purchasing Institute's ineffectiveness, Rothman was impressed by another purchasing-reform organization: The Leapfrog Group. Representatives of General Motors, General Electric, and other large companies formed The Leapfrog Group in 2000 to stimulate "giant leaps forward" in health care safety, quality, and affordability by mobilizing employer purchasing power. Its key strategies included rewarding hospitals that had strong performance data.

Rothman had good reason to be familiar with Leapfrog. Early on, its representatives had approached the Robert Wood Johnson Foundation for funding, and in response he arranged for Helms' organization to provide some of its Purchasing Institute grant money to support Leapfrog's operations. Also, several Leapfrog board members were on the Purchasing Institute national advisory committee. Indeed, Leapfrog and the Purchasing Institute had a close relationship. The staffs collaborated on some activities, and the two organizations even had a common home; in January 2001, the Leapfrog staff moved into the suite of offices within Helms' organization.

Nevertheless, the two had very different operating styles and objectives. While the Purchasing Institute was trying to improve health care purchasing through education, Leapfrog put its primary focus on pushing hospitals to initiate specific quality and safety practices, such as the use of computerized medication-ordering systems. The business executives who governed Leapfrog wanted direct action that produced measurable improvement—not training courses and reports.

By 2002, Leapfrog was growing, and seemed to be making progress toward its patient-safety goals. The organization also had a highly regarded CEO, Suzanne Delbanco, and was getting favorable publicity in the media. In short, Leapfrog was hot—and the Purchasing Institute was not. Also, some purchasing experts involved with both organizations viewed the latter as less effective. Milstein, a Leapfrog founder as well as a Purchasing Institute national advisory committee member, said in an interview that the Purchasing Institute suffered from poor leadership and a lack of oversight from above.

Leapfrog was on the lookout for more funding, and while Rothman was interested in providing it, he saw no way to justify funding both Leapfrog and the Purchasing Institute. Initially, he urged Piper and Delbanco to combine their two organizations and jointly seek Robert Wood Johnson Foundation support. Neither seriously pursued the idea. As Rothman explained it, that left him with a choice between one organization that had received lots of money but had little apparent impact and another that had little money and lots of impact.

Pulling the Plug

By early fall 2002, Rothman, after extensive consultation with his colleagues at the Foundation, came to the conclusion that the Foundation should discontinue its support of the Purchasing Institute and transfer the unused funding to The Leapfrog Group. That was the recommendation he took to the Foundation's senior management—president and chief executive officer Steven Schroeder and executive vice president Lewis Sandy—for approval. (The transfer was among the items brought to the Foundation's trustees in January 2003; Rothman said several members were consulted informally, but at the meeting itself there was no discussion of—or vote on—the action.)

While recognizing the unusual nature of ending a national program midstream, Rothman said he did not want to waste more money just because he was afraid to admit a mistake. If anything, he should have moved a year earlier, he said.

Rothman informed Helms of the closure decision on October 29, 2002. The news, Helms said in an interview, came as a surprise—and one with a significant financial impact on AcademyHealth. If the Purchasing Institute was not performing properly, the Foundation should have given him—the head of the grantee organization—a chance to fix the problem before closing down the program, he contended.

Throughout the life of the Purchasing Institute, according to Helms, Rothman had dealt with Piper. By all appearances, the two men got along well and did not need or want his involvement, Helms said. "I never heard directly from Michael Rothman about any issues related to the management of the program." Nor, Helms noted, was there any need to. "Piper was the national program director, not me," he said. "AcademyHealth was serving as the institutional home for the program." Once the Purchasing Institute included private purchasers and dropped Medicaid, he no longer felt ownership, Helms said. "I believe my concept got hijacked by the Foundation." As Helms saw it, Rothman was the program's director at the Robert Wood Johnson Foundation, and Piper, although an AcademyHealth employee, worked for Rothman.

Piper, too, was surprised by the decision. According to him, the feedback from the Foundation up until then had been positive. Giving him responsibility only a few months earlier for a new $7.5 million program, Rewarding Results, is not the signal a foundation sends if it is dissatisfied, he said. Berenson, the former CMS official and now a senior fellow at the Urban Institute, was also surprised by the closure decision. Berenson was critical of the Purchasing Institute's performance but said he viewed the

Rewarding Results grant as a sign that the Purchasing Institute must be doing what the Robert Wood Johnson Foundation wanted it to do.

The Closure Process

Although the closure decision had been made, the timing and severance arrangements were still to be worked out. For the Purchasing Institute staff, the result was a period of uncertainty and anxiety. "It was like ripping a Band-Aid off very slowly," a staff member said.

According to Helms and Purchasing Institute staff members, the Foundation's plans for the closure—or at least their understanding of the plans—kept changing. Initially, their impression was that the phase-out might last as long as a year, and that there was a good chance the Purchasing Institute staff would be able to transfer to the Leapfrog payroll. In fact, Leapfrog ended up hiring one Institute staff member, a research assistant. A second became director of the Consumer-Purchaser Disclosure Project, a position funded out of Leapfrog's new Robert Wood Johnson Foundation money.

The Purchasing Institute officially closed on the last day of February 2003. The Foundation gave Piper a transition contract to produce a series of educational materials for purchasers. Other staff received three months' severance pay. Along with the Purchasing Institute's unused funding, the Foundation transferred the Rewarding Results authorization to Leapfrog—a total of more than $4 million, according to Foundation records.

In return, Leapfrog became responsible for providing technical assistance to the Rewarding Results demonstration projects and supporting the Consumer-Purchaser Disclosure Project. Otherwise, it could use the Robert Wood Johnson Foundation money to support and expand its core activities. There was no requirement that it take over the Purchasing Institute's education-related functions.

—m— An Outside Assessment

In July 2002, the Robert Wood Johnson Foundation contracted with Mathematica Policy Research to conduct a short-term assessment of the Purchasing Institute's effectiveness. If the results were positive, the Foundation intended to commission a more comprehensive assessment, including a survey of between 100 and 200 key CMS managers and private-sector purchasers.

The original purpose of the assessment was to help the Foundation prepare for a January 2004 decision on renewing the Purchasing Institute and not for the early-closure decision in 2002, according to Foundation records. Both Rothman and Marsha Gold, who directed the work for Mathematica, said the findings had no effect on the closure decision. Nevertheless, during or shortly after that decision-making process, the Mathematica team reviewed Purchasing Institute documents, met with Piper and his staff, and interviewed fourteen individuals familiar with the program, including CMS officials and private purchasers.

In a confidential memorandum to the Foundation in November 2002, the Mathematica team listed the Purchasing Institute's principal accomplishments:

- Helping build the field of purchasing through publications and other information dissemination
- Serving as a neutral convener able to bring people together and facilitate meetings
- Providing financial and administrative support to Leapfrog and the Consumer-Purchaser Disclosure Project
- Permitting CMS to gain more knowledge of private sector activity

The memo also cited program limitations—unclear goals, lack of a substantive strategy, and weak staff expertise—and drew these main conclusions:

- "The initial emphasis on Medicare purchasing no longer dominates National Health Care Purchasing Institute."

- "From its inception, the Purchasing Institute has lacked clarity about its goals, and this continues to be a source of tension and potential conflict within the Foundation and field."

- "Unless the Purchasing Institute's mandate is restricted to facilitation, it needs to add senior technical expertise."

—∿— Issues for Consideration

The outcome of the Purchasing Institute raises at least four key questions:

1. *Program Design: Was the Purchasing Institute, as designed, capable of achieving the Foundation's goal?*

   The Foundation's Purchasing Institute experience shows the difficulty of turning one person's concept into a functioning, effective program, said Barrand, the Foundation program officer for the planning grant. The concept got lost as the initiative moved through different hands at both the Robert Wood Johnson Foundation and the grantee organization, she said.

   There is, of course, no guarantee that Etheredge's original idea—improving public-sector purchasing through exposure to private-sector practices—would have worked. David Lansky, the national advisory committee member, said the idea never made sense to him. There are legal, cultural, and other fundamental reasons that CMS does not act like General Motors, and education is not going to change them, he said.

   But adding corporate purchasers broadened the program's audience and, in the view of some observers, made progress in any one area hard to achieve. "The bottom line is that the Purchasing Institute was given a difficult charter," said Delbanco, who left her Leapfrog position in 2007. Nikki Highsmith, a senior vice president of the Center for Health Care Strategies, agreed. The Purchasing Institute's effort to reach its diverse constituency resulted in materials that tended to be generic instead of market-specific, she said. By contrast, the Center's Medicaid purchasing program—which Highsmith started—had a narrow, captive audience and, as a result, could provide direct technical assistance without bothering with glossy publications, she said.

In addition to being diverse, the target was a moving one—even after the design stage. Indeed, there is a sense that much about the Purchasing Institute got made up as it went along. The definition of its private-sector audience was initially Fortune 100 companies, but a year later expanded to the Fortune 500. Meanwhile, Medicaid purchasers dropped off altogether. As the Purchasing Institute evolved, the perception grew that it was a program mainly for corporate purchasers. Given this fluctuation, it is not surprising that the Mathematica assessment found a lack of goal clarity.

Another question is whether education was an effective strategy to improve purchasing. One lesson from the Purchasing Institute's experience, said Delbanco, is that philanthropic support for direct action to bring about change is likely to have a greater impact than support for educational efforts to stimulate change. Or as she put it, "Get one step closer to the bottom of the food chain." The Purchasing Institute had a good purpose—education—but education alone turned out to be insufficient as a mobilizing agent, Bradley said.

2. *Oversight: Would better oversight have improved the chances for success?*

As an oversight mechanism, the national advisory committee was all but nonexistent. To be effective, Lansky said, an advisory committee must have a chair and a process for bringing its advice to bear on program operations. If a foundation expects an advisory committee to be more than advisory—to actually monitor a program—it must make that expectation clear to the members, added Darling of the National Business Group on Health. Kerr, the former Ford executive who also served as Leapfrog's chair, said the lesson was that when the Robert Wood Johnson Foundation gives money, it must be clear about the expected outcome and make sure there is a measurement system in place to show if and when the outcome is achieved. In hindsight, said Rothman, he should have been more active in determining the national advisory committee's role. "I should have looked to David Helms and the national advisory committee to give more guidance."

A key element of oversight is communication, and here the Center for HealthCare Strategies saw problems on both sides. The Robert Wood Johnson Foundation signaled its dissatisfaction with the Purchasing Institute's performance, but failed to convey the seriousness of the concerns, she said. On the other hand, Piper did not react to the signals as aggressively as he should have, she said.

Communication is not necessarily just verbal. Less than a year before deciding to close down the Purchasing Institute, the Foundation gave its staff responsibility for a new $7.5 million grants program, Rewarding Results. Is that the kind of message—and money—that the Foundation should be sending to a grantee that is not performing up to expectations?

3. *Staffing: Did the Purchasing Institute have a staff fitted to the mission?*

Some observers—both inside and outside of the Foundation—questioned the strength of the Purchasing Institute's leadership. When rolling out a new program, the Foundation's usual practice is to select the director and then house the program in that person's organization. It was the other way around with the Purchasing Institute. In hindsight, should the Foundation, rather than the Alpha Center, have driven the selection of the program's leadership?

Beyond the doubts about the program's leadership, the makeup of the support staff was also open to question. By all accounts, the six or seven Purchasing Institute staff members below the director were hardworking, responsive, and competent, particularly at putting on meetings. But as several interviewees noted, none had a background in health care purchasing. They were essentially management and administrative personnel. As a result, once Etheredge and Ward left, the Purchasing Institute was largely dependent on outside consultants for purchasing expertise.

If it is to be effective, should a program that is designed to provide expertise have experts on staff? A need for senior technical expertise was one of the conclusions of the Mathematica assessment. "There are a variety of ways to enhance technical expertise. The current use of episodic, task-oriented consultants probably is insufficient," the assessment team concluded.

Another question is whether Etheredge's departure should have raised more of a red flag at the Foundation than it did. To Barrand, the lesson is that when a program suffers a major personnel upheaval, the Foundation should put operations on hold and sort out the problem before proceeding. In this case, a couple of months spent evaluating the program's goals and direction could have been beneficial, she said.

4. *Closure: Was an early shutdown of the program appropriate, and if so, could the Foundation have handled the situation more effectively?*

Certainly, Rothman's explanation for the closure—that he didn't want to waste more money just because he was afraid to admit a mistake—is hard to argue with. Nevertheless, the withdrawal of the Purchasing Institute's funding and the way the decision was carried out raise questions.

First, it is worth emphasizing that this was not a program up for renewal—the usual know-when-to-hold-'em, know-when-to-fold-'em situation. The Purchasing Institute was in the fourth year of its five-year authorization when the Robert Wood Johnson Foundation decided to transfer the unspent funding to The Leapfrog Group. The actual closure came at the end of the fourth year.

Robert Galvin, General Electric's executive director of health care services and chief medical officer and a founder of The Leapfrog Group, praised the Foundation's decision to close the Purchasing Institute as a bold move that showed the kind of flexibility private industry applauds. "I was in favor of closing the Institute," he said, "because it had served its purpose and other organizations were filling the need."

Patricia Salber, who spoke at a number of Purchasing Institute training sessions, viewed the Foundation's decision through a different lens: as a co-founder and co-president of a defunct nonprofit (Physicians for a Violence-free Society), Salber admits to being sensitive to any sign of philanthropic fickleness. The Purchasing Institute, she said, put on useful educational conferences and published high-quality educational materials. That was her understanding of its purpose. If it was supposed to do more than that—and she had no knowledge of plans for follow-up conferences and hands-on projects—she would not argue with ending the program early, she said. But if the Foundation shifted its own objective for the Purchasing Institute from education to direct action—changing the rules in the middle of the game, in her words—she questions the fairness of yanking the grant before the end of the grant period.

Either way, the Purchasing Institute episode raises questions about how to handle an early program termination. What does the Robert Wood Johnson owe the grantee organization beyond any legal requirements?

DeParle, the former Foundation trustee and CMS administrator who is now with the Obama administration, said the Foundation should follow a formal, transparent process. Before closing the Purchasing Institute, it would have been prudent to step back, fully evaluate the program, and give Helms a chance to make changes, she said. She expressed concern that the shutdown appeared arbitrary and secretive.

For the Purchasing Institute staff, closure no doubt would have been stressful however gently done. But a concrete, clearly communicated plan at the outset would have made the experience easier to take, said the two staff members who were interviewed. "They just owed us a more thoughtful process," one added.

—∽— Conclusion

Samuel Smiles, another nineteenth-century writer from the British Isles, is not as well known as Oscar Wilde, but he, too, had something relevant to say:

> We often discover what will do by finding out what will not do; and probably he who never made a mistake never made a discovery.[3]

The Robert Wood Johnson Foundation's Purchasing Institute experience offers numerous lessons about what it is likely to "do" and "not do" in philanthropic undertakings. Here are a few possibilities as a starting point:

- Maintain clarity about the objectives, the activities for achieving them, and the audience to be reached. If there is confusion or disagreement on any one of these, work it out to the satisfaction of the key players—and don't proceed until then.

- Play an active role in selecting the individual to lead an intervention, and ensure that he or she buys in fully to the planned objectives and strategy.

- When dealing in a technical area, make sure the implementing staff possesses relevant expertise.

- If conflict among key personnel becomes disruptive, call a time-out until the issue is fully understood and fairly resolved.

- Clearly identify the individual responsible for implementing the intervention and keep communications flowing with him or her.

- Establish an oversight committee that is engaged and make sure it is utilized by the funding and implementing organizations.

- Set realistic but meaningful measures of performance and effectiveness and ensure that the necessary measurement data is generated and collected.

- If an initiative proves to be ineffective, give the responsible individual a chance to take corrective action.

- If a program cannot be salvaged, don't be afraid to end it prematurely, but do so in an orderly, transparent way that allows affected staff to understand the situation and have reasonable time to find other work.

Notes

1. Wilde, O. *Lady Windermere's Fan*. Project Guttenberg, 1997. http://www
   .gutenberg.org/etext/790. Accessed on June 10, 2009.
2. See the Robert Wood Johnson Foundation. "Borrowing Business Practices to Improve Medicare." *Grant Results Report*, March 17, 2003.
   http://www.rwjf.org/pr/product.jsp?id=17023. Accessed on June 10, 2009.
3. Smiles, S. *Self-Help*. London: John Murray, 1876.

The Role of Failure in Philanthropic Learning: A Commentary on Chapters 1–3

Robert G. Hughes

T he three preceding chapters share the theme of examining Foundation efforts that did not achieve their desired ends. In a word—failure.

In the first of the three, Stephen Isaacs and David Colby draw on eight programs that "didn't work out as expected" to illustrate three reasons that programs do not succeed: strategy or design flaws, challenging environments, and faulty execution. Tony Proscio identifies three similar reasons in his chapter, this time applied to the need to redesign programs in midcourse. He delves into two case examples of programs changed in midstream—SmokeLess States and Supporting Families After Welfare Reform. He complements these two real examples with a third, composite case created from a number of programs to convey real problems and choices while preserving the anonymity of the people involved. In the third chapter, Mike Brown offers a detailed case study of one program that was terminated early, the National Health Care Purchasing Institute. Overall, these chapters present a nice array—eight programs that, in retrospect, didn't work; two programs (and a program composite) that were recognized as not working at the midpoint and were redesigned; and one program that was not working and was closed early. In combination, these three chapters provide an important milestone in the Foundation's longstanding practice of assessing its own performance and publicly sharing the results.

—⌇— The Importance of Learning from Failure

The uniqueness of philanthropy is built on its independence—its relative freedom from systematic market and public account-ability constraints. This oft-noted feature of the philanthropic sector undergirds the sector's rich diversity of approaches and is the source of much of its influence. But the societal and institutional benefits of this relative autonomy for individual foundations—in diversity of approaches, independence of think-ing, and innovation—are balanced, when it comes to judging effectiveness, by relatively weak relationships between foundations and the environments in which they operate. Feedback loops are attenuated, and the capacity for constructively critical commen-tary is undermined along two dimensions: the assessment of a foundation's performance and a foundation's assessment of the environments in which it operates. This leads to two important challenges:

- Developing and sustaining a framework for assessing the performance of foundations
- Designing ongoing mechanisms for scanning environ-ments and using that knowledge strategically

Both challenges respond to the autonomy that characterizes an independent foundation and its environment. The first can be viewed as looking at a foundation "outside in"; the second can be viewed as looking "inside out." Both underscore the value of interaction with the environment to generate better performance. For foundations striving to be learning organizations, these two challenges are central. Learning organizations need critical judgments to improve.

As a learning organization* committed to continual improvement, the Robert Wood Johnson Foundation values both assessments of its performance and insights derived from analyzing the environments in which the Foundation works. Failure and success represent the ends of a continuum of judgments about performance, so they are critical conceptual anchors for addressing the challenges above.

What is the status of activities that respond to the two challenges? The first challenge—assessing foundation performance—has garnered much more attention than the second. Indeed, the second is often completely neglected. Yet even regarding the first challenge, where progress *has* been made recently, the Center for Effective Philanthropy, which is leading the call for comparative assessment of performance of foundations, indicates that the field has much room for growth.[1]

Foundations are attempting to judge their own effectiveness in a variety of ways, from evaluations to balanced scorecards. Trends in philanthropy such as striving for greater transparency, clarifying goals, and specifying logic models reinforce the movement toward better performance assessment. Yet progress is not speedy. At the Robert Wood Johnson Foundation, assessing performance has been an important element of its culture since it became a national foundation in 1972. Indeed, in their chapter, Isaacs and Colby posit that the Foundation "is widely considered as being in the forefront of learning from its programmatic experiences" and

---

* A learning organization for our purposes is an enterprise that is committed to improving through structured thinking about its performance relative to its environments and its goals.

"is striving to develop a culture whereby the staff and board learn from the results of its programs, both positive and negative." Yet there is an intriguing end to that sentence: "though Foundation staff members candidly confess that there is a long way to go." What explains the implication that to learn from programs, especially those with "negative" results, is so difficult?

We know that organizational learning in general is hard.[2] In foundations, it is especially so. Proscio's description of a pivotal moment in the case study of Supporting Families After Welfare Reform helps explain this. He notes that for a program officer armed with a critical evaluation of the program's first year performance, "it would not have been unusual . . . to remain upbeat and noncommittal." He goes on: "Instead, he chose to deliver the news unvarnished." The program officer noted that "it was unusual to have that kind of conversation." We can learn two things from this. The first is to appreciate the individual courage required to share negative judgments about performance. The second is the pervasive, deep-seated aversion to critical assessment such that, even in an institution that values such judgments, unvarnished bad news is unusual.

This leads to the question: why is it important to use the word "failure?" It is precisely because foundations are among society's freest institutions—their influence and relative autonomy allow them to avoid confronting failure—that they should push themselves to be rigorously honest about how they are doing, including their failures. Foundations seeking to improve their performance need critical assessments of their performance—to "confront the brutal facts," in the phrase of Jim Collins, author of *Good to Great*.[3]

This is an ongoing effort at the Robert Wood Johnson Foundation; these three chapters show that progress is being made, but it takes a great deal of care and effort. Insight into why it is so difficult can be found in the reasons that led Proscio to use a "composite" case in his chapter. As Proscio notes, these cases involve people and their lives and careers, and contained disagreements and disappointments; it is painful to have these publicly discussed. Failure is tough to talk about—it is not a popular topic, and we tend to avoid it if we can. And if a foundation's culture reinforces, rather than counteracts, that understandable inclination, the likelihood of confronting the brutal facts is even less.

Isaacs and Colby "have chosen to avoid the word 'failure' since even programs that do not work as expected can provide valuable lessons and directions for the future." I agree that programs that fail can serve those important learning functions, but I depart from my colleagues in avoiding the word "failure." In fact, using the word "failure" is especially important in philanthropy precisely because it is so easy to avoid.

Along with staff members from eight other foundations, in 2008 I participated in an Action Learning Group organized by Grantmakers for Effective Organizations that explored the topic: Leveraging "Failures" in Philanthropy. One of the biggest challenges faced by the learning group was, in my judgment, dealing directly with the idea of failure. Discourse about failure does not come naturally to the field, indicated even in the quotation marks around failure in the group's task. Yet acknowledging failure is essential to learning and improving performance in any field. Charles Bosk documents how the best surgeons are those who can acknowledge their own mistakes.[4] In philanthropy, failure has been almost invisible until the last few years.[5]

Compare learning in philanthropy with learning in the sciences. Scientists must hold two potentially conflicting positions simultaneously—passionate belief in their hypothesized explanations and eagerness for objective evidence to test those beliefs. In one sense, philanthropy is similar to science. Philanthropic programs, especially those intended to be strategic, are hypotheses about how the world works, and they test what will happen if a program is implemented successfully.

But philanthropy's incentives reward program staff for generating hypotheses much more than for seeing what happens. In language familiar to foundations, Isaacs and Colby observe that "program officers are motivated largely by the development of new and exciting programs. Once a program is conceived and approved, it is easy to forget it and move on to the next." Although this apparent imbalance in institutional incentives has little influence with some staff members, its effects are reflected in Isaacs and Colby's observation that "many foundation staff members are tempted to oversell a program to get its approval."

These tendencies to focus primarily on program development and grant making to the neglect of implementation are challenged by the constellation of activities that aim at assessing organizational performance and using that information to improve performance; that is, learning. And failure is an important window to organizational learning.

—∿— Approaches to Thinking about Philanthropic Failure

Failure has only recently become a focus of interest in philanthropy, but it has many possible applications. This section maps out some initial approaches to analyzing failure that may be useful as a framework for future discussion. The initial focus, in keeping with the first challenge to foundations, is on failure and performance assessment of programs. This is followed by an exploration of how failure fits into the second challenge for foundations—understanding their environments.

Failure and Performance Assessment

In the context of the performance of a foundation, failure can be viewed from three perspectives: the reasons for failure, levels of analysis, and stages of program life cycles.

Reasons for Failure

Both Isaacs and Colby's chapter and Proscio's chapter examine why failure happened and produce three broad categories: difficult environment; strategy or design flaws; and faulty execution. While not using the same terms, much of Brown's in-depth case study reinforces the utility of these categories, and gives texture to how, in practice, all three may contribute to a program's failure. The three reasons for failure provide a useful high-level framework for thinking about the main components of programs and their performance. Indeed, one benefit of this analysis of failure is the utility of the framework for assessing successful programs as well. Proscio's chapter on midcourse corrections suggests a possible fourth reason for failure that is implicit in his cases: a failure to adapt.[6] Proscio notes the powerful forces that resist midcourse corrections. Adding failure to adapt as a fourth category would emphasize the importance of ongoing assessment to program effectiveness and provide an antidote to the perceived institutional incentives that favor program development and grant making over implementation.

Levels of Analysis

Common to all three chapters is the level of analysis. Failure can occur at many different levels, and the choice for analysis is an important one. A simple taxonomy (beginning with the most basic level) could be project, program (cluster of related projects), major initiative (cluster of several programs focused on the same topic), and field (cluster of major initiatives around a strategic goal). Language in philanthropy is notoriously vague, and institutions often develop their own vocabulary, so let me quickly acknowledge that this particular taxonomy may not be useful across foundations. The point is that activities with a purpose occur at different levels, and being clear about the level is important for two reasons.

First, the field appears to put disproportionate attention and resources toward assessing the performance at the lowest level (projects) and very little attention to assessing high-level strategies. Arguably, the priorities should be reversed. For example, Patrizi

Associates' analysis of field building in end-of-life care from 1996–2005 is an extremely valuable but rare example of a high-level assessment.[7] The predominant pattern of attention on the lowest level—projects—inhibits an understanding of how projects fit together over time and relate to the environment in which they operate. In turn, this reinforces a focus on a project's internal risk—implementation—and away from strategic and design risks. Note that failure of implementation puts the spotlight on grantees; failure of strategy and, to some extent, design puts the spotlight on foundations.

Second, there is an unfortunate tendency to use grants or monetary transactions as the starting point for analysis. The starting point for assessing performance—including understanding failure, success, risks, and strategy—should be the desired end, whatever the level of analysis. Grants are tools that may correspond to a project, or not. For example, the analysis of the National Health Care Purchasing Institute is organized around the purpose of the Institute, and this set of activities was supported by multiple grants to different institutions. The purpose guides the analysis; the number and composition of the grants is secondary. While grants are sometimes crafted around desired ends, that is not necessarily the case, and to start with grants in order to assess performance is a significant disadvantage. Beginning with grants also reinforces the perspective that the work of a foundation is making grants, rather than reaching goals. Indeed, one indication of a foundation's ability to assess its performance is the ease with which it can organize such assessments around desired outcomes rather than financial transactions.

Stages of Program Life Cycles

Almost all philanthropic programs have a time horizon and a related life cycle—development, implementation, conclusion. Performance assessments can be conducted for each stage. The development stage is a primary focus of program staff, as they aim to develop programs that the Foundation will fund. Looking only at this stage, failure is a decision by the Foundation not to fund the program.

The examples of failure explored in the three chapters are all of programs that were successful in the first stage, that is, they all received funding through the decision-making process of the Robert Wood Johnson Foundation. Nevertheless, they shed light on the decision-making process. For example, at least some knowledgeable observers would have expected Community Programs for Affordable Health Care (CPAHC) to fail, even before the decision was made to fund it. This was not the case for SUPPORT. Note the difference in the reactions to program failure—with CPAHC, there was criticism of the basic model from knowledgeable experts. With SUPPORT, those in the field were stunned; they were surprised that the intervention failed, since it had been crafted by leaders from the field itself. Thus, an important difference in these two failed programs could have been the testing of the feasibility of the hypothesis before the decision was made to authorize the program. One of the most promising new developments for philanthropy is the application of new Web 2.0 tools to gather a wide array of views about a proposed strategy, as The David and Lucile Packard Foundation did with its "nitrogen wiki."[8] Packard used a wiki, a social media tool that solicits ideas from a broad audience, to obtain input on its new strategy to reduce nitrogen pollution. Opening the process of developing program strategy through tools such as wikis potentially decreases the likelihood of the kind of failure that CPAHC experienced.

Failure and Environmental Assessment

A second, much less developed approach to the uses of failure is in exploring the capacity of foundations to scan and understand their environments. This second approach implies a basic shift in orientation. The first approach—performance assessment of program work—takes a goal or strategy as a given and asks why a program fails or succeeds. It is at heart an internal orientation. The second approach—environmental assessment—begins with the environments in which a foundation operates; it starts with the context from which the goals and strategies are developed and within which they are carried out. It is at heart an external orientation, looking outside the boundaries of a foundation and its programs. This orientation raises a different set of questions around the relationship of foundations to their environments, beginning with such basic ones like:

- What are the environments in which foundations operate?
- How do foundations analyze their environments?
- How do foundations look at risk?
- How do foundations think about their role relative to other actors in the environment?
- Where do program ideas come from?
- How do foundations expect program activities to be sustained in future environments?

Foundations operate in two related environments: the world of philanthropy and the world defined by their mission—in the case of the Robert Wood Johnson Foundation, health and health care. This is a basic but often overlooked feature of a foundation's context. It suggests that, at a minimum, there are two types of learning, each based on potential successes and failures, which foundations should consider. *Philanthropic learning* is about understanding and improving the craft of philanthropy and the various ways it can be conducted. *Mission-related learning* is different. It is about understanding and improving the fields in which the foundation operates. For the Robert Wood Johnson Foundation it is about improving health and health care, often at the level of programs.

As an example of the two types, take the Foundation's contribution to the emergence and establishment of the country's 911 system in the 1970s.[9] The Foundation-funded Emergency Medical Services program was evaluated for its performance in the field of health care, and the results were published by the National Academy of Sciences. Commissioning independent assessments and supporting their publication in scientific reports or peer-reviewed journals is common practice for the Foundation. Yet these outlets are in the fields in which the work was conducted. They are not even on the radar screens of the philanthropic world. Once they are put into a field's journal, such as *Health Affairs,* that field becomes the lens for understanding the work. So any lessons for grant making that might be derived from such assessments are often overlooked.

One possible implication of the different learning environments in which a foundation operates is in the design of knowledge-management systems. The lessons drawn from a foundation's experience in a mission-related field (such as improving health and health care) are largely connected to that field's learning more broadly, and thus should be communicated through vehicles such as Web sites and publications targeted to the field. Philanthropic learning—that is, learning related to grant making and other approaches used by foundations—has both an internal (staff) and external (foundation colleagues and interested public) audience, so mechanisms for sharing that knowledge should be designed to accommodate both.

Foundations could benefit from going beyond simply being aware of their environments to analyzing them and their potential risks, and using the analyses in future planning. At the Robert Wood Johnson Foundation, we have used the Monitor Group and GBN—firms with expertise in specific approaches to environmental scanning—to help explore the context of our future work. This scanning has been done for the Foundation as a whole as part of its overall long-range strategic thinking and for its individual program portfolios. Each portfolio has a distinctive approach to producing social change, a different time horizon, and a different tolerance for risk. The different purposes and risk tolerances lead to expectations for different kinds of learning as well, including types of success and failure. The Foundation's pioneer portfolio, for example, which seeks to identify ideas and practices with breakthrough potential for the future of health, has a much higher tolerance for risk, and thus for certain types of project failure, than the human capital portfolio, which identifies and trains future health and health care leaders.

Focusing on environments highlights a foundation's role relative to others in the field and stimulates thinking about how these relationships could be structured to further the foundation's objectives. Understanding a foundation's role relative to that of other actors is a critical (and ongoing) step in determining, in a disciplined way, what a foundation can and cannot do. The Boston-based Barr Foundation, for example, has adopted an approach that relies on the various systems within which its works takes place, and it sees its role as a part of those systems. "We work at 'mapping' and tracking these systems and identifying the numerous ways in which they intersect, influence each other, and change over time," The Barr Foundation writes. "Understanding the dynamics of these systems and partnering and collaborating with the key players in them are central to our ability to identify effective 'levers' for sustainable change."[10]

Another example is the Gates Foundation, which explicitly depends on other actors to achieve progress in reaching its goals, downplaying the relative importance of its own grant making in furtherance of the collective effort. Shifting to a network or multi-stakeholder framework triggers a different conceptualization of how performance assessment—including judging success and failure—is approached. The lack of a rigorous environmental assessment that clearly defines areas of program opportunity increases the risk of redundancy and decreases the likelihood of program effectiveness.

Thinking about the environment can help foundations focus on two additional questions, both related to programs: Where do ideas come from? What happens when a program is over? Recognizing that ideas seldom originate from the Foundation helps staff members to appreciate the valuable roles of people and organizations in the field in generating ideas. It is in the identification of promising program ideas and practices that social media hold great potential for foundations. The Robert Wood Johnson Foundation has used online idea competitions through Changemakers, a program of Ashoka, as part of program development. These competitions simultaneously produce new ideas, connect social entrepreneurs to a like-minded community, provide an efficient, fast overview of work on a topic, and provide the field with a framework that shows where there is progress and where there are gaps that need attention.

At the other end of the life cycle of a program, an internal, rather than outward, orientation—one that focuses primarily on strategy and execution of programs—often neglects sustainability issues until near the end of a program. For example, the two largest philanthropic supporters of the end-of-life field— the Open Society Institute and the Robert Wood Johnson Foundation—withdrew their funding from the end-of-life field at about the same time, slowing the considerable momentum that had been achieved. Understanding the environment could help foundations address issues of sustainability and avoid unnecessary difficulties.

—⁓— Conclusion

Foundations derive their influence from their relative freedom and unencumbered resources, which provide the underpinning for their potential to bring new ideas to life. Yet with the freedom and resources comes a critical responsibility—to do this work as effectively as possible, and to get better at it over time. How does the field, or a particular foundation, get better? One promising approach is by looking at foundation performance through its relationships with its environments, and learning from failures. Overall, critical and honest examination of their work will help foundations become more realistic about their impact and more effective at fulfilling their contributions to society.

Notes

1. Center for Effective Philanthropy. *Indicators of Effectiveness: A Call for Foundations: Understanding and Improving Foundation Performance*, 2002. http://www.effectivephilanthropy.org/images/pdfs/indicatorsofeffective ness.pdf. Accessed on June 10, 2009.
2. Schein, E. H., and Coutu, D. L. "The Anxiety of Learning." *Harvard Business Review*, March 2002, 2–8; Garvin, D., Edmondson, A., and Gino, F. "Is Yours a Learning Organization?" *Harvard Business Review*, March 2008, 109–116.
3. Collins, J. C. *Good to Great: Why Some Companies Make the Leap—and Others Don't*. New York: Harper Collins, 2001.
4. Bosk, C. *Forgive and Remember: Managing Medical Failure*, 2nd ed. Chicago: University of Chicago Press, 2003.
5. Gilroth, R., and Gewirtz, S. "Philanthropy and Mistakes: An Untapped Resource." *Foundation Review*, Winter 2009, 115–124.
6. I first came across this idea in a staff paper by Steve Downs and Chinwe Oneykere in a 2003 analysis of risks for the Foundation's pioneer portfolio.
7. Patrizi, P., Thompson, E., and Spector, A. "Death Is Certain, Strategy Isn't: Assessing RWJF's End-of-Life Grantmaking," presented at the Strategy Forum of the Evaluation Roundtable, May 21–23, 2008.
8. Kasper, G., and Scearce, D. *Acting Wikily: How Networks Are Changing Social Change*. Monitor Institute and David and Lucile Packard Foundation, 2008.
9. See Diehl, D. "The Emergency Medical Services Program." *To Improve Health and Health Care: The Robert Wood Johnson Foundation, 2000*. San Francisco: Jossey-Bass, 1999.
10. Barr Foundation, http://www.barrfoundation.org/about/index.html. Accessed on June 10, 2009.

Section Two
Inside the Robert Wood Johnson Foundation

5. Communications at the Robert Wood Johnson Foundation:
   Turning Up the Volume, Adjusting the Frequency

Communications at the Robert Wood Johnson Foundation: Turning Up the Volume, Adjusting the Frequency

Frederick G. Mann and David J. Morse

Editors' Introduction

The Robert Wood Johnson Foundation's communications strategy has evolved dramatically over the past few years. From the very beginning, the Foundation has been strategic in its grant making, and its first staff members knew that reaching its strategic goals would require the adoption of an approach that Frank Karel, the Foundation's vice president for communications between 1974 and 1987 and again between 1993 and 2001, called "strategic communications."[1] These are, in Karel's words, "communications activities creating information and effecting the exchange of information tailored to foster relationships and actions crucial to advancing the Foundation's mission and goals."[2] Karel was the pioneer of strategic communications in foundations, and this approach has characterized the communications work of the Robert Wood Johnson Foundation ever since. As a core element of that approach, the Foundation downplayed its own role, choosing instead to speak through its grantees.

This strategy was appropriate in its day. Times have changed, however, and beginning in 2003, the Robert Wood Johnson Foundation began to articulate the idea that it was in the business of fostering social change and that this could be done most effectively by advancing public policies that better promote health and health care. Around the same time, communications technology began to explode as the Web took off, e-mail became the norm, and search engines such as Google cranked up their power. The changes in the Foundation's approach to policy and the arrival of new information technologies led it—perhaps even forced it—to reconsider its communications strategy and make adaptations that would make it appropriate for the times.

David Morse, the vice president for communications at the Robert Wood Johnson Foundation, and Fred Mann, the assistant vice president for communications, were the chief architects of the new communications strategy. In this chapter, they present an insiders' view of why it was necessary to develop a new strategy, how the strategy evolved, what its main elements are, and what challenges remain. It is one of those *Anthology* chapters that explore the inner workings of the Robert Wood Johnson Foundation and share them with a broader public. Since the Foundation is widely considered to be in the forefront of philanthropic communications, this chapter will be of particular interest to leaders and communications officials of foundations and other nonprofit organizations as well as to those charged with developing strategic communications policies and programs, wherever their place of employment.

Notes

1. Karel, F. "Getting the Word Out: A Foundation Memoir and Personal Journey." *To Improve Health and Health Care: The Robert Wood Johnson Foundation Anthology, 2001*. San Francisco: Jossey-Bass, 2001.
2. Ibid.

I t's not easy to build on the work of a master. Oh, sure, a lot of the heavy lifting has been done for you, and many of the pivotal early battles have been won. But trying to follow in the large footsteps of a well-known leader in any field is a difficult mission at best.

In our case, the field is foundation communications, and the leader whose vision we are attempting to keep current and adapt to changing times is Frank Karel, longtime vice president for communications at the Robert Wood Johnson Foundation and at the Rockefeller Foundation, former program officer at the Commonwealth Fund, former journalist, and, in the eyes of many, the man who almost single-handedly raised the stature and the strategic importance of communications throughout the foundation world.

Back in 2001, just before he retired (for the second time) from the Robert Wood Johnson Foundation, Karel wrote for this *Anthology* series about how our foundation's communications efforts had evolved over the years.[1] "Foundations have been slower to integrate communications into their institutional planning and work than any other class of organizations in our society," he wrote. Commenting on the congressional hearings leading up to passage of the Tax Reform Act of 1969—sweeping legislation that affected the operation of private foundations, many of which had taken a public beating, he noted: "The prevailing mood and mindset in the foundation world was to keep as quiet and as low a public profile as possible."

Karel set out to change that mindset. He brought a modern sense of communications to this foundation and others, and he helped put strategic communications planning and practice in the center ring of philanthropic work. "Communications has become an integral part of everything we do," he wrote in his 2001 *Anthology* chapter. "The aim is to share our vision of using communications strategically—that is to create and use information in ways that can help achieve key organizational and program objectives."

We have tried to build on Karel's firm footing and, as he did, align communications efforts with the Foundation's objectives. But as those objectives and strategies have evolved over the years, so, too, has our approach to communications. Today our programs focus largely on influencing and changing public policy and organizational practice to improve the health and health care of all Americans. The key tools we use for influence are advocacy, public education, and communications. We advocate for change. We inform policy debates. We have more targeted and time-delineated goals focused on bringing about positive improvements in people's lives. Our big-issue approach to improve health care quality, to reverse the childhood obesity epidemic, to build and fortify public health systems, and to provide affordable and stable health insurance coverage for all has made influencing public policies and systems vital to us.

"It is through policy change that societies make and remake themselves," the Foundation's senior vice president for health, James Marks, and the journalist Joseph Alper wrote in their chapter "Shaping Public Policy as a Robert Wood Johnson Foundation Approach" in Volume XII of this series. "With limited philanthropic resources available, working to change policy offers foundations the possibility of improving the lives of many more people than they could through other forms of grant making, such as direct services grants. And the improvements are likely to be longer lasting since once enacted, policy remains and becomes part of the societal landscape. For foundations, this represents social change and one of the most effective ways they can leverage their investments."[2]

Today the Foundation has a voice in the policy arena. And we want that voice to be heard. Our megaphone is our new communications model—a direct descendant of Frank Karel's "getting the word out" approach, but now a more strategic, centralized, policy reform-focused system that does more than just complement our programmatic objectives; it is essential to actually bringing about the lasting social change we seek.

Of course, as Frank Karel noted, cranking up the communications volume and effectiveness does not come naturally in the foundation world. Foundations can be quiet places. Ours certainly often seems to be.

Foundation staff members don't sell product or maximize revenue. Instead, their fundamental purpose is to make a difference in people's lives. As far as work with a purpose goes, this is at the top of the scale. You'd think the people who got to do this would be singing and dancing and throwing confetti on the way out the door each night. But that's not foundation culture. People at most foundations do love their work and know that the impact they have to improve the lives of others can be huge. But the workplace is usually dignified, polite, scholarly, not showy or boisterous. When Rebecca Rimel, the president and CEO of The Pew Charitable Trusts, was once asked by a visitor why her foundation was so quiet, she replied, "Yes, we're a bit like ducks you see gliding quietly and effortlessly across a pond, but if you look just below the surface, you see those webbed feet paddling furiously. So it's quiet at the surface, but not so quiet below."

Still, it seems pretty quiet in areas where communications officers congregate. Their counterparts in print, broadcast, and online newsrooms may celebrate a great series with high fives and war whoops (and a truly notable achievement like a Pulitzer Prize with sprayed champagne), but foundations and their communications staffs are far more circumspect. As Joel Fleishman noted in his insightful 2007 book *The Foundation: A Great American Secret*, "Foundations have generally shared a 'culture of diffidence' that discourages openness about their activities and agendas."[3] This diffidence, he writes, stems in part "from a long-prevalent sense that it is unseemly for a charitable giver to 'toot his own horn' by publicizing his gifts. For many tradition-minded philanthropoids, even issuing press releases about their grants feels uncomfortably like bragging."

So imagine the odd scene the morning of April 4, 2007, when the staff of the Robert Wood Johnson Foundation gathered around a large projected image of their president and CEO Risa Lavizzo-Mourey—and cheered her appearance on NBC's *Today* show. She was there to promote the Foundation's very public announcement that it would devote $500 million over the next five years to reverse the nation's dangerous childhood obesity epidemic.

The announcement went far beyond the comfy couches of *Today*. As envisioned in a plan drawn up by Adam Coyne, the Foundation's director of public affairs, the *New York Times* carried a lengthy exclusive story about the Robert Wood Johnson Foundation's ambitious childhood obesity pledge; the Associated Press wrote a story that ran in scores of papers around the country; Lavizzo-Mourey and other Foundation representatives appeared on the nightly network news shows, PBS's *NewsHour with Jim Lehrer,* NPR (National Public Radio), and other key news outlets.[4] The Foundation laid the groundwork by sending information on the Foundation's commitment to more than 800 reporters covering health, health care, and philanthropy; distributing a video package to more than 200 television and radio stations nationwide; updating the Foundation Web site; posting an electronic letter to more than 25,000 grantees and Web site content subscribers; and contacting every member of Congress, every governor and lieutenant governor, mayors in the 100 largest cities, members of state legislatures' health committees, and federal agencies and organizations.

—⚘— The Way We Were and Why We've Changed

Given Frank Karel's strong guidance, the Robert Wood Johnson Foundation was never particularly shy when it came to communicating. Under Karel's leadership, the Foundation's communications department grew in both size and mission. Communications became integral to Foundation programs, and communications staff people were full members of Foundation program teams. Communications-related grants, largely for the Campaign for Tobacco-Free Kids to reduce smoking among teens and for ads produced for the Partnership for a Drug-Free America, grew significantly, and accounted for more than 20 percent of all funds awarded by the Foundation from 1997 to 2001.

But even as communications took a central role within the Foundation, the messages reaching the outside world could be somewhat scattered, and sometimes even contradictory. For most of the Foundation's history, our explicit approach to communicating about mission, goals, strategies, and objectives had been that "we speak through our grantees." That approach was expressed a decade ago by then-president Steven Schroeder in a statement of core values and commitments. But even as he affirmed this grantee-centered communications strategy, Schroeder noted drawbacks to the approach—that speaking indirectly through many grantees who themselves have different objectives made it more difficult for the Foundation to "influence the policy process" and that "we pay a price in the potential attenuation of policy leverage."

Our influence in shaping change in health and health care, therefore, has been derivative historically, since our grantees were our principal agents who executed Robert Wood Johnson Foundation strategies. Having multiple voices delivering multiple messages on different issues (or even the same issue) was harder for key audiences to process than sending consistent messages from consistent sources. Furthermore, when the Robert Wood Johnson Foundation spoke about an issue—like health insurance coverage, tobacco, or end-of-life care—primarily through grantees, it was difficult for those receiving messages to know the overarching goals and objectives of the Foundation, the nature of its role and relationship to a grantee, and the salience of the issue to the Foundation, policymakers, and the public.

Grantee-centered communications made perfect sense when the Foundation was initiating and funding national programs and projects that were loosely related to one another within broadly defined fields: access; quality; addiction prevention; healthy communities and lifestyles—its goal areas in the 1990s and early 2000s. But today our programming is more targeted, giving way to a drive for measurable social change in policy, in organizational practice, and in behavior. In 2003, Risa Lavizzo-Mourey assumed the presidency of the Foundation and developed an "Impact Framework," which continues to guide our programs to this day. This framework organized the Foundation's philanthropic investments through a set of diversified portfolios, much like those of mutual funds, to meet short-term, medium-term, and long-term goals. This structure has brought a sharp focus to how we try to solve pressing health and health care problems, and has also given us the means to more effectively manage and measure the results of our work.

The Impact Framework also required a different approach to communications—one that emphasizes the Foundation's speaking collaboratively *with* our grantees and other colleagues in addressing the issues that are the pillars of the framework—like the need for health coverage for all Americans and rolling back the tide of childhood obesity. Rather than embedding communications resources directly in each major grant, with each grantee communicating independently, we have shifted our communications approach to intentionally speaking together and collaboratively *with* our grantees rather than *through* them— viewing grantees and the Foundation as an interdependent family of people and programs with common goals and common messages.

Communications dollars that used to be included in grants so that grantees could independently promote their work and publicize their findings and their accomplishments are now largely held back and are spent at the Foundation level. Instead of grantees issuing statements and releasing white papers that could step on the toes of other grantees working in the same field, messaging and timing of communications is now coordinated centrally by the Robert Wood Johnson communications staff. The result is greater efficiency and, we believe, greater impact.

As we took these steps—centralizing communications strategy and messaging, speaking collaboratively with grantees, tying communications objectives closely to our philanthropic program goals—we were doing something new and unlikely for us: putting ourselves in the spotlight along with our grantees. Not because we sought more ink but, rather, because we sought a paradigm shift in the conventional wisdom about philanthropy generally and the Robert Wood Johnson Foundation's philanthropy specifically: to accelerate and accentuate a shift in perception from simply being a *grant maker,* or provider of funds for good works, to that of a catalyst, expert, and leader in creating systemic change and improvement in health and health care.

In a 1998 *Health Affairs* article, Steven Schroeder not only restated his "we speak through our grantees" philosophy but also added, "(we) do not seek a high institutional profile. We have chosen to work primarily through our grantees, rather than establish ourselves as a primary source of information." A decade later, we and our grantees firmly believe that we can have a greater collective impact if the Foundation speaks and stands *with* them rather than speaking *through* them.[5]

The strategy for maximizing our communications impact is fairly simple. First, create common, closely aligned communications on behalf of issues that we, grantees, and colleagues are addressing together—like rolling back childhood obesity, creating greater quality and equality in health care, and improving the health of vulnerable people by attacking the social factors that impede their health. Second, link these communications across programs and issues into a more comprehensive approach, one that we hope is a more robustly influential Robert Wood Johnson Foundation in which the whole is more than the sum of the parts.

Enhancing our influence as a health and health care leader and leveraging our impact fully requires us to speak more authoritatively as a foundation, to strengthen our credibility as a source of essential information about changing policy and practice, to attract significant and influential partners, to add value to our grantees' work and reputation, and to elevate our stature as a guiding force and catalyst for change in health and health care.

—ᴠᴠ— It Began with a Promise

Discovering the benefit of building our own image and speaking directly for causes we champion was not a quick or easy process. It started with the idea of identifying the Foundation's brand—what the Foundation was and why we were in the business we were in. As long ago as 2002, President Schroeder brought together twenty-five staff members from all levels of the organization, along with a few members of the Foundation's board of trustees, to ascertain the characteristics of our Foundation's brand. To even consider that a philanthropy had a brand was unprecedented: brands were seen as the province of the corporate world, and of large nonprofit organizations that provided direct benefits, like education, health care, and social services. We had a mission statement, well-articulated goals, and a tag line (most often heard on NPR), but we didn't have, or didn't think we had, a brand.

At Schroeder's five-hour evening meeting, people sat at a large, open-square table, each with a laptop computer, for what Dave Richardson, president of Wirthlin Worldwide (now Harris Interactive), the lead facilitator of the session, called an Advanced Strategy Lab. Richardson started by describing what a brand and branding were: "management of actions and communications with constituents to move them from what they *currently* think of your organization to how *you want them* to think of the organization." In other words, according to Richardson, branding is about being known for attributes *we* (the organization) would like *you* (our audience or constituents) to know about. He then peppered the group with questions. Each person entered brief answers on a laptop, and then viewed their collective responses almost immediately on a large screen at the front of the room.

His first question was simple: "What business are you in?" The dominant answer was simple, too: "We're in the grantmaking business." Richardson paused and asked the question again: "What business are you in?" Again the same answer. But he clearly expected a different response, so he asked a slightly different question: "Is grant making the *purpose* of your business or is it *what* you do?"

You could almost see the collective light bulbs going on in the heads around the room, and could see them literally on the screen at the front: "Aha, we're in the social change business— the business of improving health and health care for all Americans. Grant making is what we do—a means to our goals, not why we do it."

It was clear that the group, all insiders, considered the Robert Wood Johnson Foundation to be essentially a bank or a philanthropic ATM machine—you put your card in, in the form of a grant application and, after some due diligence, you got your money (or not, if your application was turned down). And that was conventional wisdom about foundations, from both inside and outside the philanthropic world—that we were essentially *transactional* organizations.

That was certainly the way the public—through the prism of the press—saw us. A recent survey by InfoTrend of 40,000 news stories mentioning foundations since 1990 showed that 99 percent of those stories were about transactions—grants made or paid—and not about foundations' or even their grantees' impact.[6]

Recognizing that the transactional brand we thought we had wasn't the one we wanted to have was hard. In 2002 and 2003, we organized similar branding labs with grantees, representatives of media organizations, and policy leaders. Ironically, they understood that the Foundation's mission was about catalyzing social change in health and health care better than the Foundation staff who participated in that first lab. They recognized that our greatest asset was our reputation for objective data, building evidence, and creating influence for change, not simply the dollars we provided.

And then we conducted the labs with the entire staff, and finally developed a set of characteristics that reflected, we think, both what the Foundation was and what we aspired to be. It reflected more about what others thought of us and what we should be than what we had thought of ourselves. But we still couldn't call it our brand, since that would be too "commercial," according to most of the staff. We called it the Robert Wood Johnson Foundation Promise.

Moving from a principal mindset of being basically a grant maker to seeking impact and influence in health and health care hasn't been without challenges, and it hasn't happened overnight.

The Robert Wood Johnson Foundation Promise

We care deeply about the pressing health and health care issues that this country faces. When issues of national magnitude—like covering the uninsured, improving the care of chronic illnesses, developing the next generation of leaders, improving the health of the most vulnerable among us, revamping our public health system—need leadership, the Robert Wood Johnson Foundation has traditionally stepped forward.

The reason isn't simply that significant issues need significant resources. For 35 years, we've brought not just our financial assets, but our deep experience, commitment and a rigorous, balanced approach to the problems that affect both the health care and the health of all those we serve.

We focus on issues that demand attention. We work with a diverse group of people whose dedication, expertise and perspective lead to sound, new solutions. We will not shy away from difficult or controversial questions. And we have the staying power to stick with problems until solutions become clear, momentum has been established, and progress has been made.

We believe in supporting programs that have measurable impact and that create meaningful and timely change—helping Americans lead healthier lives and get the care they need—because we expect to make a difference in your lifetime.

It took two years before we could even consider moving from using the "Promise" euphemism (although it's not a bad one) to using the "B" word. But there is increasing comfort, among both staff and grantees, with the concept of a Foundation brand and, more importantly, with its implementation. Results in 2008 from our annual "Scorecard" survey of health experts, business leaders, and policymakers suggest that these key Foundation constituencies resonate with core characteristics of the Robert Wood Johnson Promise. They believe that the Foundation addresses important, difficult issues in health and health care; that we stick with addressing long-standing problems; and that we're objective and rigorous.[7]

—∿— A Culture of Storytelling

We think, as did Frank Karel, that the best way of getting the word out about the Foundation, our grantees, and our collective impact is by telling stories about our work and about the people we are trying to serve. As our colleague Andy Goodman describes in *Storytelling as Best Practice,* while evidence—the "cold hard facts"—is critical to making one's case, it's the story, supported by evidence, that convinces and moves one to action. In his introduction to Goodman's monograph, Ira Glass, the founder and host of public radio's *This American Life,* a mecca for storytelling, notes "The most powerful thing you can hear, and the only thing that ever persuades any of us in our own lives, is [when] you meet somebody whose story contradicts the thing you think you know. At that point, it's possible to question what you know, because the authenticity of their experiences is real enough to do it." Richard Wirthlin, the communications guru and adviser to Ronald Reagan, a consummate storyteller, put it more simply: that people are persuaded rationally but motivated emotionally.

Goodman, a Foundation grantee, thinks so: "To evaluate how well an organization communicates, I start by looking at how well it tells stories about its work. I don't care how big they are or how many resources they have at their disposal—if they can't tell a good story, then they haven't mastered the most fundamental form of human communication." He notes that the Robert Wood Johnson Foundation is developing a culture of storytelling, and, even better, insisting that its grantees do so as well. "Now, this doesn't mean that Robert Wood Johnson doesn't rely on data to make its case; like most foundations, it is awash in numbers," he says. "But its program officers and staff use stories as the spear point to pierce the veil of apathy (or distraction, or the numbness of information saturation) and get their audience's full attention. And once they have that attention, then they present the data to show there is more than one story to be told."

—∿— Measuring Up

"The Robert Wood Johnson Foundation today understands that communications means more than just publishing a report. It is really about creating a simple, compelling message that can get people to change their behavior," says Bruce Siegel, a physician who is the director of the Center for Health Care Quality at the Department of Health Policy at George Washington University School of Public Health and Health Services. "Sometimes this means targeting patients, other times nurses or CEOs. But it is still about helping someone to understand that they need to do things differently."

Siegel, a former New Jersey commissioner of health, who has served as the director of several Robert Wood Johnson Foundation national programs, says that the Foundation's staff members "work hand in glove with their expert partners to understand a problem as well as its solutions. Then they seek to use the entire array of media to spread a consistent message that can move people to action. A big part of this process is absolute honesty: the goal here is to figure out what really works, not just what makes us feel good about ourselves."

But how do we know what really works? How will we know if we have really done our job well? How do we measure progress toward our goals? In certain instances, measuring the success of a communications effort is pretty easy. Take the childhood obesity announcement. We had newspaper clips to read and television news tapes to watch. We saw traffic on the Foundation's Web site spike to new levels, and we had phones ringing off the wall with calls from people eager to help us spend the $500 million we had pledged. But without clear and precise strategic programming and communications plans to spend that huge sum of money wisely and effectively, a raised Foundation profile is just an easy target at which critics will shoot.

Our program team working on reversing the childhood obesity epidemic by the year 2015 has those strategic plans—and more. For example, it is actively pushing for policy changes on the national, state, and local levels that will improve the nutritional quality of food served in schools, reinstate physical education, and improve the access to affordable fresh food and safe places for children to play in poor and vulnerable communities. They are funding studies, convening experts, and creating a new hub of knowledge and action for the field in the Robert Wood Johnson Foundation Center to Prevent Childhood Obesity. With the new center, they are helping to create an online community that will serve as the go-to resource for our major community-based action and advocacy programs, *Healthy Kids, Healthy Communities,* and *Communities Creating Healthy Environments,* as well as our other grantees and the obesity-prevention field at large. There is substance backing up the $500 million public pledge.

"The legitimacy and persuasiveness of a foundation's voice in its efforts to influence public policy depends entirely on the evidence-based knowledge and carefully-researched program demonstrations with which it can buttress its views," says Joel Fleishman, author of *The Foundation* and professor of Law and Public Policy at Duke University. "Unless backed up by evidence that persuades, a foundation's voice is just another person's opinion. What infuses the Robert Wood Johnson Foundation's communications efforts with great credibility are the thirty-eight years of consistent devotion to finding out and documenting the extent to which its grantmaking initiatives have indeed been effective, and to sharing its findings with the professional community and the public. That honesty and that openness are what give great weight and influence to the Robert Wood Johnson Foundation's efforts to persuade the public, the policymakers and the relevant professions."

Not all communications efforts, however, are as clear to measure—or so certain to have impact or be noticed as having impact—as pledging to give away $500 million.

If you're in the business of being a philanthropic bank, measurement of success seems fairly simple: numbers of grants made, dollars out the door to meet annual required payout, geographic and demographic distribution of grant funds—all can be counted. But if you're in the business of measuring social change, outcome seems far more complex. What's the marginal contribution of a foundation, a grantee, or any other single organization to driving down smoking rates among America's youth, increasing enrollment of eligible kids in the State Children's Health Insurance Program, rolling back the national epidemic of childhood obesity, or improving the quality and equality of health care in, say, Cleveland or Memphis? And can we measure the contribution and the cost-effectiveness of our communications efforts toward those goals? Since we're a health foundation, we often think in the language of prevention and treatment—what's the right formulary and dose of communications to reach a particular goal?

One of our goals over the years has been to ensure that all Americans have affordable, stable health care coverage. There are more than 46 million uninsured people in the United States. With our Foundation's assets, we could probably buy an inexpensive, high-deductible health insurance policy for a few million uninsured Americans for a year. That's easily measurable—but we wouldn't have a foundation anymore. So we've focused on increasing the salience and the political and economic unaccept-ability of having 46 million uninsured in America. For several years, we have mounted a series of Cover the Uninsured cam-paigns, with partners like the American Hospital Association, the AFL-CIO, the United States Chamber of Commerce, America's Health Insurance Plans, and others[8]—all organizations that rec-ognize that we can't sustain a society in which tens of millions have no access to high-quality affordable care, but all of which have very different perspectives on how to address the problem of uninsurance.

The campaigns are intended to help change the frame—the perceptive boundary—in which the public, opinion leaders, and policymakers know and understand who the uninsured are. Understanding who they really are, we believe, can increase the propensity of policymakers to act on their behalf. We've done market research, conducted polls and focus groups, tested and retested messages, done pre- and post-campaign analyses. Since these campaigns began, the dominant frame has changed. The research tells us that the public no longer sees the uninsured as simply the downtrodden looking for a handout, but, rather, as people like *you*—parents and kids in working families, your close relatives, your neighbors and friends—who aren't uninsured by choice but because they or their employer can't afford insurance. Americans now know that 80 percent of the uninsured are in working families.

Is that a communications success? While the fundamental goal of stable, affordable coverage for all Americans is still elusive, we seem to have achieved what we believe to be one of the build-ing blocks toward reaching that goal. But what's our foundation's marginal contribution toward creating a new conventional wis-dom about the uninsured? We've asked an outside evaluator—a political scientist at the University of Minnesota—to help us answer that question. He will report back to us in a few months.

Some communications professionals say it's okay to measure "contribution rather than attribution." A former boss calls it "plausible connectivity"—a reasonable link between what we sought to do and the desired outcome, even if there's a lot of noise in the system that makes it difficult, if not impossible, to tease out the marginal contribution. Perhaps. But we are still searching for that magic measurement bullet.

By one measurement, it appears as if our new communications approach is reaping benefits. According to a content analysis of articles in the top twenty-five American newspapers, long-lead magazines (like *Time* and *Newsweek*), and health trade journals, of 1,400 articles reviewed between 2003 and 2008 that mention the Foundation, 26 percent (370) associated the Robert Wood Johnson Foundation with specific brand attributes—our leadership, strategies, partnerships with key players, policy aims and outcomes—rather than simply transactions. (It's a nice improvement over the InfoTrend study showing 99 percent of stories about all foundations being strictly about transactions.) This analysis, conducted by CARMA International, states that the brand attributes most associated with the Foundation were leadership, making a positive difference in people's lives, successful partnerships, policy influence, and taking a strategic approach to meeting its mission. These data reflect media coverage in only a few specific, albeit important, print media—not broadcast, cable, Web, and other electronic and social media that we know are increasingly where the general public and opinion leaders connect and get their information. But we view the print content analysis as a positive sign not just that our Foundation messaging is being heard but also that we seem to be growing our impact and influence.

—⁓— Growing Electronically

Our main vehicle for sharing information about impact is our Web site and the electronic media strategy that undergirds it. Like many other foundations, we are aligning our communications model to take advantage of the new interactive features and functionalities that social media and Web 2.0 technologies provide. Foundations have never been early adopters, but they have been using Web sites to promote their grantees and their work for many years. Now, with the growth of social media, those sites have the capacity to be much more than promotional vehicles and online storage rooms for white papers and grantee reports. Today's technology is all about interactivity. The Web site is not just the Foundation's front door to the world; it is the home for debate, dialogue, creation, and connection for both the foundation and its audiences. And, happily, it is one form of communications outreach where participation (if not clear success) is measureable.

It's fair to say that back before we changed our communications model and started to see how a Web site could really build a connection with key audiences and give us a larger voice, our site wasn't as good as it should have been. RWJF.org was hard to navigate, and users found it hard to search for information they wanted and knew was there. There was no clear indication of our priorities; the audiences we particularly wanted to reach—policymakers, opinion leaders, the media, as well as our current and prospective grantees—would have a hard time figuring out what we, the Foundation, thought was most important. Our program teams were more focused on making and managing grants than on collecting and promoting the learning and knowledge gleaned from their work. The Web site was considered the exclusive province of the Foundation's Communications and Research and Evaluation units.

Since the change to the team-oriented Impact Framework approach and the embracing of the Robert Wood Johnson Foundation brand, program staff members now understand that their role extends beyond just grant making. They have increasingly turned to using the Web site and related electronic media to drive toward meeting team objectives and promoting the learning derived from our philanthropic investments. But despite this important internal conversion—and some good trends that showed a steady growth of our online audience—we were still not doing enough with the Web. One of our program teams, the one working to improve both the quality and equality of health care, was eager to embrace the Web in order to build interest in its issues, share results, and interact with all sides of the health care quality debate. But given the technical and design constraints of RWJF.org, the team could not see the Web site filling its new needs.

So at the end of 2007 we embarked on a quick but thorough redesign of the Foundation's Web site to enhance our impact, promote social change, and showcase the knowledge and experience that are core elements of the Foundation's brand. We also did it to take advantage of all of the benefits that the expanding interactive Web offers. In June 2008, in conjunction with the announcement of the Foundation's $300 million investment to improve quality in health care markets in specific regions across the country, and guided by a new cross-Foundation Editorial Policy Board that sets Web strategy and oversees the quality and focus of our electronic communications products, we re-launched RWJF.org. Its target audiences remained policymakers, policy influencers, state officials, congressional staff, grant seekers, grantees, and the media. And what they found was a site that was more flexible—more able to spotlight goals and developments like the regional health care quality effort—and fresher and newsier, with content changing more frequently to drive repeat user traffic.

We improved the design of the Web site to better display both the programmatic work of our teams and, in keeping with our new higher profile approach, to show the Foundation's commitment to social change. We improved the site's search and navigation functions so that our large volume of reports, analyses, and evaluations could be more easily found by our Web audience. On the new RWJF.org, visitors can more quickly and easily learn what the Foundation is about and what we deem important. They can continue to receive weekly "news digests" about issues and events in childhood obesity, nursing, health insurance coverage, and other key fields, and timely "content alerts" highlighting new developments in research and policy related to public health, vulnerable populations, and quality and equality of care.

In early 2009, with health reform becoming a major issue of interest in Washington, we launched a new Health Reform section of our Web site. The section continues to grow and serves as a home for comprehensive, balanced, timely information on important reform issues with content being provided not only by Robert Wood Johnson but also by other responsible news sources and by active participants on our health reform blog.

Information across the site is now presented in forms that are easier for Google and other search engines to find and display. Our new internal analytics capacity helps us follow site usage patterns in detail. We can determine who is coming to RWJF.org, where they are coming from, how long they are staying, which reports and publications they are downloading, which program areas and subfields have the most loyal following, and how many visitors are signing up for our news digests and other electronic products.

Knowing how many policymakers and other information seekers are coming to us and what they are interested in is an important measure of the effectiveness of our communications outreach and our programming work. Our editorial policy board and Web team are tracking various metrics carefully to learn what types of content are most valued by our different audiences.

The new Web site also provides the social media functionality we knew we needed, which allows for greater information sharing and collaboration with grantees and users. We are currently hosting blogs, discussion boards, and interactive chats. We have established a Robert Wood Johnson Foundation presence on YouTube, Twitter, and soon Facebook—the most ubiquitous Web-based social-networking channels. We have syndication (RSS—Really Simple Syndication) feeds available on hundreds of topics and publication types so people can get automatic feeds delivered to them on topics of their choice. And we are integrating these feeds into grantee Web sites. We are crawling their sites for content we want to display on the Foundation's site, and we are exporting our content to our grantees' sites via "widgets" (pre-branded headline components that allow the Foundation to offer news digests, the latest research and publications, news releases, and other content, sorted by topic.) We have also built a "Slidebuilder" in order to easily present charts and Power-Point presentations from grantees; congressional, state and local policymakers now are able to download or print them easily and include this Foundation content in their presentations and reports. This has answered a clear need, particularly for our policymaker audience and for others who wanted quick, digestible, graphical information.

We have created a central grantee product repository that allows us to collect publications from our grantees and display them both internally for our staff and externally on RWJF.org. In short, we are building a content distribution network that will turn the Foundation and our major grantee sites into one family with all our knowledge products given maximum distribution, all on behalf of the specific social changes in health and health care we and our grantees and philanthropic colleagues seek—rolling back childhood obesity, securing health care coverage for all Americans, transforming our outmoded public health systems, and improving the quality and equality of care. It's less about tooting our own horn and more about influencing these transformative goals.

—∿— Connecting with Policymakers

One indication that policymakers are starting to take more notice of your stature in the field is how often they ask not for your money but for your advice. The Robert Wood Johnson Foundation is unique among American foundations in having a formal program to link the Foundation and our grantees directly and strategically with policymakers in Washington and increasingly in the states. It's called the Connect project, and through it the

Foundation's leadership and our grantees have become sources of congressional testimony and expert advisers on health and health care matters.

Connect was founded back in 1998 by the ever-forward thinking Frank Karel and one of his communications officers, Joe Marx. It was designed to help our grantees establish and build relationships with their congressional delegations. Of course, the Foundation is prohibited from lobbying, and our grantees are prohibited from using our funds to lobby. But Connect is not about lobbying—it's about educating members of Congress and their staff about the critical health challenges and creative solutions being developed, tested, and implemented in their states and districts. It's about engaging policymakers to learn about and support these promising projects in non-legislative ways: through site visits, with letters of support, and by connecting grantees to key partners in the community.

Since its inception, Connect has scheduled meetings between hundreds of Robert Wood Johnson grantees and their members of Congress, and has organized dozens of Capitol Hill briefings for congressional staff members to highlight the work of our grantees. Over time, the program has also incorporated a robust training element to ensure that grantees are well-prepared with a clear message, a compelling story, and a specific, non-legislative "ask" in each of their meetings, and has provided technical assistance to grantees to ensure that they follow up on those asks effectively when they go back home.

Although a Robert Wood Johnson representative typically accompanies the grantees on their meetings with members of Congress and their staff, and usually leaves behind a list of Foundation-supported projects in the member's state or district, Connect has been solely focused on positioning the grantees—and not the Foundation itself—as resources on the Hill.

As the Foundation shifted its communications approach to speaking *with* our grantees, the Connect project expanded its focus. Although we continue to support our grantees through training, meetings, and briefings on Capitol Hill, we also began, in 2006, to have a more explicit focus on positioning the Foundation itself as a resource to federal policymakers and their staff. Several times each year, senior staff, including our president and CEO (and, occasionally, our board chair) meet with members of Congress both to share our lessons learned and to seek advice from the leaders in Congress on health and health care. These meetings allow us to put the work of our grantees in a broader context and to make connections across the Foundation's program areas.

Reaching out to members of Congress and developing relationships with them and their staff has led to additional opportunities for Robert Wood Johnson Foundation staff members to testify at congressional hearings, in some cases alongside our grantees. For example, in October 2007, Risa Lavizzo-Mourey testified at a House Energy and Commerce Health Subcommittee hearing on tobacco; a Foundation grantee, William Corr, then executive director of the Campaign for Tobacco-Free Kids, was also a witness. In 2007 and 2008, Foundation staff members testified at congressional hearings on childhood obesity, quality, and disparities in health care. Working with the Connect project, Foundation grantees have also testified at hearings on long-term care, school nutrition, and childhood obesity.

Not all of our Connect work is done in Washington. For instance, in 2008, after Foundation communications and program officers provided information to a *Wall Street Journal* reporter about one of our projects—Green House, an innovative alternative to a traditional nursing facility—and a glowing page one article was published, Connect organized a site visit for congressional staff members to a Green House facility. A bipartisan group of House and Senate staff members, as well as staff members from the Congressional Research Service and the Centers for Medicare and Medicaid Services visited the Lebanon Valley Brethren Home in Palmyra, Pennsylvania. There they toured the traditional nursing home on campus, as well as one of the four Green House homes on site to see firsthand the difference in the two settings, and to hear from the home's residents and staff, as well as the national program staff of the Green House initiative. Green Houses, they were told, provide an environment in which residents receive nursing support and clinical care without the care becoming the focus of their existence. By altering the facility size, interior design, staffing patterns, and methods of delivering services to residents, the Green House model provides residents with greater health and lifestyle benefits than do traditional nursing and assisted-living buildings. Early results show that Green House residents report higher satisfaction levels, less physical decline, and less depression.

The visitors heard from Robert Wood Johnson staff members about the Foundation's support for the Green House, and also about our broader commitment to improving long-term care and community-based services for the nation's aging population. Through visits such as this, people making public policy get the opportunity to see the work of Robert Wood Johnson and its grantees and come to understand the role the Foundation can play in helping Americans lead healthier lives and get the care they need.

—⁓— Plans for the Future

Expanding Connect is but one way we hope to keep moving forward with communications efforts aimed at fostering policy change. Through greater content sharing with grantees on the Web and co-branding of grantee and Foundation products electronically and in print, we seek to broaden the distribution of our knowledge and spread awareness of how we can influence policy debates. Our goal is to continually make our communications collaborative, not derivative. Among our specific goals for the next few years are these:

Expand Our Outreach to News Organizations

Establishing a voice for the Foundation is one thing. Having that voice heard is quite another. Robert Wood Johnson was an early foundation supporter of NPR, starting back in 1985, and has continued its support for health reporting from 1986 through the present day. In addition, the Foundation has, since 2005, funded health reporting on PBS' *The NewsHour with Jim Lehrer*, which has been ranked first among all television news programs as the most credible, objective, and influential. The survey further notes that *The NewsHour* is among the leading programs in reaching elite policy makers who directly affect a broad range of health issues.[9] By supporting strong journalism that increases the scope, the quality, and the depth of health and health care reporting, important policy issues are most effectively raised to a more engaged public and to policymakers. For the past ten years, we have also been a major supporter of the Association of Health Care Journalists, feeling that members of this organization are also well-positioned to provide accurate, timely news and analysis on issues of importance to the Foundation and its target audiences. These connections help raise the Foundation's profile with journalists and, through them, with health and health care decision makers.

In 2008, we took another large step in supporting quality journalistic coverage of issues important to us by giving a grant to Columbia University's Graduate School of Journalism to underwrite the health and science portion of its new one-year master of arts journalism degree program. To be called the Robert Wood Johnson Foundation Program in Health and Science Journalism, it will train young and midcareer journalists to bring depth to their coverage of health and science, and provide students with specialized knowledge and a sense of context and history. The public and policymakers need reporters and editors who can effectively explain and compellingly present complex issues of health and health care.

The Foundation is coordinating with Columbia to ensure that curriculum development broadly reflects the goals and interests of the Foundation. We also will invite students to come to Princeton to meet with program and communications officers working in their fields of interest, and Robert Wood Johnson Foundation staff members will periodically travel to Columbia to speak and to provide guidance and expertise. Students in the program will become Robert Wood Johnson Foundation Fellows in Health and Science Journalism. As part of the Foundation's scholars and fellows programs, this cadre of journalists will enrich our alumni network and strengthen the Foundation's impact on the future of health and health care in this country. Not incidentally, we hope our grant also helps promote our influence with health and health care journalists.

Reach Outside Mainstream Media

Many of the key audiences and constituencies we serve—those most affected by childhood obesity and by inequities in quality of care, our most vulnerable populations, the nation's diverse group of health workers and professionals—go outside mainstream media channels for credible information. At the same time, many journalists working for media outlets serving specifically ethnic or culturally based audiences often say that health coverage is a major priority for the communities they serve. These newspaper, magazine, broadcast, and Web outlets are deeply interested in receiving culturally relevant health information from credible organizations. For many such publications and programs, their role goes beyond simply informing their audience; they also help empower people and are leading voices for change in their communities. African American and Hispanic journalists in particular often see themselves as activist participants in, rather than merely observers and reporters about, their communities. They've told us that they're interested in covering some of the Foundation's key areas of work, such as disparities, access to care, obesity, and prevention. We believe we are well positioned to provide the pipeline of information that these journalists, producers, and managers need and desire.

Serving various multicultural groups with quality health and health care information will not be an easy task. Aside from a few powerhouse entities like Univision and Spanish-language wire services, multicultural media outlets tend to be small-scale and fragmented across a wide array of ethnic subgroups and narrow geographic locations. Even so, we have supported them, both through our national program, Sound Partners for Community Health, and through a series of grants to Radio Bilingue in Fresno, California.[10]

Multicultural media journalists with whom we interact, especially at Spanish-language outlets, express a strong preference for diverse spokespeople, since the audiences for such media place greater value on hearing from experts from similar racial, ethnic, and cultural backgrounds. We currently do not have a large pool of Foundation or even grantee spokespeople to draw upon for this purpose. And there is a growing interest in data and research that is specific to multicultural audiences and their needs. In other words, they are looking for targeted news they can use from people they know, can trust, and speak their language both literally and culturally.

By focusing staff attention and resources to serve ethnic and culturally based audiences with important health information, we will significantly increase the impact of Foundation programs among key populations while also infusing the Foundation's organizational culture with the appreciation that working with diverse audiences is a default tactic, not a special project.

The days of the low Foundation profile—of hiding our light under a bushel—are gone for us because they have to be gone. We can best aid in the accomplishment of our targeted, policy-change goals through speaking out directly and collaboratively, not staying in the background anymore. We are far from mastering this new on-stage role. Sometimes we are not aggressive enough in getting our messages out. Sometimes our internal processes slow us down and we miss opportunities to have an impact. Sometimes we still get tangled up with grantees who are not quite singing the same song we are. But in general we think our updating of the communications model takes us in the right direction—a direction of which Frank Karel would approve. It's a model that fits the needs and the goals of the modern Robert Wood Johnson Foundation—even if it doesn't always fit with quiet foundation culture and our inherent modesty and wonkiness.

Notes

1. Karel, F. "Getting the Word Out: A Foundation Memoir and Personal Journey." *To Improve Health and Health Care: The Robert Wood Johnson Foundation Anthology, 2001*. San Francisco: Jossey-Bass, 2001.
2. Marks, J. S., and Alper, J. "Shaping Public Policy as a Robert Wood Johnson Foundation Approach." *To Improve Health and Health Care: The Robert Wood Foundation Anthology, Vol. XII*. San Francisco: Jossey-Bass, 2009.
3. Fleishman, J. L. *The Foundation: A Great American Secret*. New York: Public Affairs, 2007.
4. *The NewsHour* and National Public Radio are grantees of the Robert Wood Johnson Foundation.
5. The Robert Wood Johnson Foundation. *2008 Assessment Report: Tracking Organizational Performance*, December 2008. http://www.rwjf.org/files/research/3632rwjf.publicscorecard081211.pdf. Accessed on June 10, 2009.
6. Philanthropy Awareness Initiative. *The Challenge*. http://www.philanthropyawareness.org/challenge.php. Accessed on June 10, 2009.
7. The Robert Wood Johnson Foundation. *2008 Assessment Report: Tracking Organizational Performance*.
8. The following organizations have been partners in the Covering the Uninsured campaigns: the US Chamber of Commerce, AFL-CIO, Healthcare Leadership Council, AARP, United Way of America, American Medical Association, National Medical Association, American Nurses Association, Families USA, Blue Cross and Blue Shield Association, America's Health Insurance Plans, American Hospital Association, Federation of American Hospitals, Catholic Health Association of the United States, Service Employees International Union, National Alliance for Hispanic Health, the California Endowment, W. K. Kellogg Foundation, Giant Food LLC, the Kroger Co. Family of Pharmacies, Pfizer Inc., Stop & Shop, the

Amateur Athletic Union, the National Association of Chain Drug Stores (NACDS).

9. Erdos & Morgan. *Opinion Leaders Study, 2008/2009, 2009.* http://www.erdosmorgan.com/sr/ols.html. Accessed on June 10, 2009.

10. Diehl, D. "Sound Partners in Community Health." *To Improve Health and Health Care: The Robert Wood Johnson Foundation Anthology, 2001.* San Francisco: Jossey-Bass, 2001.

Section Three
Addiction Prevention and Treatment

Editors' Introduction to Section Three

Addiction Prevention and Treatment

In 1993, Michael McGinnis and William Foege, two of the nation's leading physician-researchers, published a seminal article on the actual causes of death in the United States.[1] Roughly half were attributable to what people ate and drank and how they lived their lives. Smoking, drinking, unhealthy diet, and lack of exercise were among the top contributors to death. Despite the evidence that changing these behaviors and lifestyles would lower mortality and save the country money, the United States spends relatively little on promoting good health and preventing illness.

For a long time, the Robert Wood Johnson Foundation, too, failed to address the underlying causes of death. That began to change in 1991 when the Foundation made reducing substance abuse among young people one of its three priority areas, targeting three substances in particular: tobacco, alcohol, and illicit drugs. This led, ultimately, to the Foundation's decision in 1999 to split its grant making into two, with roughly half going to improving health care and the other half to improving health (including prevention and treatment of addiction to tobacco, alcohol, and drugs). Since 1991, the Foundation has invested $1.3 billion in addiction prevention and treatment.

The following three chapters address different aspects of the Foundation's work to address addiction to drugs and alcohol. Its efforts to reduce smoking have been examined extensively in previous *Anthology* volumes.[2]

In chapter 6, James Bornemeier, a New York City-based writing and editing consultant and former journalist for the *Los Angeles Times* and *Philadelphia Inquirer,* presents the broad history of the Foundation's efforts to address addiction to drugs (as distinct from addiction to alcohol).* Bornemeier, as the author of a similar wide-ranging review of the Foundation's efforts to curb smoking in an earlier *Anthology*,[3] is well suited to write this chapter. He found that although there are some similarities between the Foundation's grant making in tobacco and drug addiction, its work to curb drug addiction lacked the long-term strategic focus and impact that characterized its tobacco work. Bornemeier concludes the chapter by exploring the reasons why the one (tobacco) was effective and the other (drug addiction) was less so.

In chapter 7, Sara Solovitch, a California-based freelance writer and former columnist for the San Jose *Mercury News,* examines the Reclaiming Futures program. This program, which the Foundation began funding in 2001, aimed at bringing about "system reform" in ten communities by developing a coordinated approach to dealing with youthful offenders addicted to alcohol or drugs. Solovitch explores the rationale for and key elements of Reclaiming Futures, the way it was carried out at three sites, and the major findings of the evaluation. Based on the evaluation's findings, in 2007, the federal government, the Kate B. Reynolds Foundation, and the Robert Wood Johnson Foundation funded Reclaiming Futures programs in fifteen more communities.

The final chapter in this section—chapter 8—shifts the focus to alcohol abuse, in the form of binge drinking on college campuses. In it, Lee Green, a California-based freelance writer and journalist, tells the story of the College Alcohol Study and of Henry Wechsler, the Harvard researcher who developed and conducted the series of surveys that make up the College Alcohol Study. Wechsler popularized the term "binge drinking," and in doing so generated a storm of controversy. For its part, based on findings from the College Alcohol Study, the Robert Wood Johnson Foundation funded the A Matter of Degree program, which attempts to make it harder to obtain alcohol on or near college campuses. It also funded the Center on Alcohol Marketing and Youth at

---

* Many Foundation-funded programs addressed addiction to both alcohol and drugs, and the two could not be disentangled. When this happens, Bornemeier examines the program in its totality.

Georgetown University, which tries to curb beer and liquor marketing aimed at college-aged students and other young people.

Notes

1. McGinnis, J. M., and Foege, W. H. "Actual Cause of Death in the United States." *Journal of the American Medical Association*, 270, 1993, 2207–2212.
2. Bornemeier, J. "Taking on Tobacco." *To Improve Health and Health Care: The Robert Wood Johnson Foundation Anthology*, Vol. VIII. San Francisco: Jossey-Bass, 2005; Montaigne, F. "The Smoke-Free Families Program." *To Improve Health and Health Care: The Robert Wood Johnson Foundation Anthology*, Vol. XI. San Francisco: Jossey-Bass, 2008. Diehl, D. "The Center for Tobacco-Free Kids and the Tobacco Settlement Negotiations." *To Improve Health and Health Care: The Robert Wood Johnson Foundation Anthology*, Vol. VI. San Francisco: Jossey-Bass, 2003; Orleans, C. T., and Alper, J. "Helping Addicted Smokers Quit." *To Improve Health and Health Care: The Robert Wood Johnson Foundation Anthology*, Vol. VI. San Francisco: Jossey-Bass, 2003. Kaufman, N. J., and Feidan, K. L. "Linking Biomedical and Behavioral Research for Tobacco Use Prevention." *To Improve Health and Health Care: The Robert Wood Johnson Foundation Anthology, 2000*. San Francisco: Jossey-Bass, 2000; Gutman, M. A., Altman, D. G., and Rabin, R. L. "Tobacco Policy Research." *To Improve Health and Health Policy: The Robert Wood Johnson Foundation Anthology, 1988–1999*. San Francisco: Jossey-Bass, 1999.
3. Bornemeier. "Taking on Tobacco."

CHAPTER 6

The Robert Wood Johnson Foundation's Efforts to Combat Drug Addiction

James Bornemeier

T he searing effects of drug addiction have always held an unrelenting attraction for Hollywood filmmakers. From 1955's *The Man with the Golden Arm*, in which Frank Sinatra's character Frankie Machine battles his demons, to Steven Soderbergh's Oscar-winning direction of *Traffic* in 2000, in which Michael Douglas plays a conservative Ohio judge devastated by his daughter's addiction to cocaine, the dark personal failures of drug abusers appear on screen as familiar, grim cinematic archetypes. While such sentiments may reflect much of the public's attitude toward drug abuse, researchers, scientists, practitioners, and treatment providers in the drug addiction field have come around to a very different point of view in the past fifteen years. Largely gone is the perception of drug abusers as flawed individuals whose decisions are to be pitied and condemned. In its stead is a consensus that drug addiction is not only a public health issue but also an issue of personal health—a chronic disease whose treatment should parallel that of diabetes and asthma.

Since the Robert Wood Johnson Foundation was established, in 1972, it has invested more than $450 million to combat the harmful effects of drug addiction. And, just as the drug abuse field at large has evolved, the Foundation's approaches have followed a similar path since the early 1990s, when it stepped up its grant making in the area.

Early efforts were aimed at seeding and cultivating a field of research—and a new wave of researchers—to undertake a range of scientific inquiry into substance abuse that had barely existed before. The goal was to develop evidenced-based findings that would be the basis for sound policy formation. The Foundation also experimented with different strategies for combating drug abuse, including the establishment of community coalitions, support of research and researchers, creation of a research and advocacy unit based at Columbia University, and support of organizations providing technical support to policy makers and service providers.

Realizing that early engagement with young people was a key preventive tool, the Foundation teamed up with Head Start to try to stave off drug abuse in high-risk settings and funded initiatives that sought to reform the juvenile justice system to better screen, counsel, and treat young people with drug problems. A long-running relationship with the Partnership for a Drug-Free America helped place thousands of TV and prints ads in an attempt to raise young people's awareness of the dangers of drugs and encourage parents to discuss drug abuse with their children.

In the early 2000s the Foundation, taking advantage of scientific findings on addiction and the brain, launched initiatives based on the model of addiction as a chronic disease, and focused on improving the treatment process. Other programs sought to strengthen the relationships between state substance abuse agencies and treatment providers.

Table 6.1. Addiction Prevention and Treatment Programs Over $1 Million Funded by The Robert Wood Johnson Foundation

	Start Date	End Date	Funding
Fighting Back: Community Initiative to Reduce Demand for Illegal Drugs and Alcohol	08/01/1988	04/30/2003	$68,000,000
CASA: National Center on Addiction and Substance Abuse at Columbia University, New York	06/15/1991	10/31/2007	$56,000,000
Join Together: A National Technical Assistance Project for Substance Abuse Initiatives	9/01/1991	4/30/2010	$41,000,000
Free to Grow: Head Start Partnerships to Promote Substance-Free Communities	05/01/1992	4/30/2007	$13,000,000
CADCA: Community Anti-Drug Coalitions of America	10/01/1992	10/31/2008	$13,000,000
Partnership for a Drug-Free America	11/01/1992	11/30/2009	$56,000,000
Substance Abuse Policy Research Program	08/01/1994	12/31/2009	$66,000,000
Bridging the Gap: Research Informing Practice and Policy for Healthy Youth Behavior	08/01/1997	11/30/2012	$58,000,000
Innovators Combating Substance Abuse	05/01/1998	06/30/2007	$7,000,000
Developing Leadership in Reducing Substance Abuse	05/01/1998	12/31/2006	$5,000,000
Reclaiming Futures: Communities Helping Teens Overcome Drugs, Alcohol and Crime	11/01/1999	12/31/2013	$30,000,000
Paths to Recovery: Changing the Process of Care for Substance Abuse Programs	11/01/2001	12/31/2008	$9,000,000
Resources for Recovery: State Practices that Expand Treatment Opportunities	08/01/2002	09/30/2006	$3,000,000
Advancing Recovery: State/Provider Partnerships for Quality	12/01/2005	06/30/2010	$12,000,000

No other foundation has played such an expansive role in combating addiction to drugs in the past two decades. But the Foundation's legacy is debated within the Foundation and without, and questions linger. Did it have a strategic plan? What were its major accomplishments? Was the decision, made in 2006, to remove addiction prevention and treatment as a Foundation priority area the appropriate one?

Perhaps the most intriguing question revolves around a body of work that is widely seen as among the Foundation's most successful: its strategy to reduce smoking, particularly among young people. What was different about the two—combating addiction to tobacco and to drugs—and what lessons can be drawn from the way the Foundation approached them?

What follows are snapshots of the major Foundation drug-addiction programs and an assessment of their overall impact. Having made more than 1,300 grants addressing drug addiction, in whole or in part, the Foundation has surely been a giant, but how in the coming years will its effectiveness be judged?

—〜— Funding Research, Cultivating Leaders

As the Foundation moved into the substance abuse field, it was clear that developing a body of solid evidenced-based research— and a cadre of researchers to carry it out—would be a priority. In thinking about research, the Foundation took a broad view and realized that working in the complicated field of substance abuse, including drug abuse, required a diversity of viewpoints to tackle its kaleidoscopic nature. That realization would prove to be one of its most important contributions to combating drug addiction.

Two federal agencies, the National Institute on Drug Abuse (NIDA) and the Substance Abuse and Mental Health Services Administration (SAMHSA), were the major sources of research funding, and the Foundation entered into an informal partnership with them. "With drugs, we had federal partners, and that was a mixed blessing," recalled Steven Schroeder, who became president of the Robert Wood Johnson Foundation in 1990. "Our federal partners had a lot of money, but they also had ideology. We knew that needle exchange would be a really good way to halt the transmission of HIV in drug abusers. But it was off limits politically. So there were certain constraints working with federal partners, but there was tremendous potential to expand the dollars and the influence."

While the Foundation's financial contributions were minuscule by comparison, it played a significant role in the drive to amass a growing body of policy research aimed at addiction. "Most of our funding was for evidence-based practices and activities, but the Robert Wood Johnson Foundation has been able to address more cross-cutting issues that influence how policies are shaped in the United States," said Jack Stein, the director of the Division of Services Improvement in the Center for Substance Abuse Treatment at SAMHSA. "It was the perfect public and private partnership. The Robert Wood Johnson Foundation was able to support a number of efforts that were out of our jurisdiction, and they enhanced work at NIDA and SAMHSA that we literally did not have the resources to do."

The Substance Abuse Policy Research Program

In 1991, not long after Steven Schroeder became the Foundation president, the board of trustees adopted as one of its three goals "to promote health and prevent disease by reducing harm caused by substance abuse." To guide its prospective grant making relative to this new goal, the Foundation needed to amass evidence-based research on which to build its programs. In January 1992, the board approved $5 million over two years to establish the Tobacco Policy Research and Evaluation Program. Two years later, it expanded the program, renamed the Substance Abuse Policy Research Program (SAPRP), to include alcohol and illicit drugs and authorized $12 million over three years to carry out research under it.[1] With subsequent authorizations, the Foundation has committed $66 million to SAPRP. (In the spring of 2009, the program stopped issuing grants; its research projects run through 2011.)

SAPRP focuses on analyzing public and private policies aimed at reducing the harm caused by substance use and abuse. It has developed the field of substance abuse policy research by supporting peer-reviewed research to increase understanding of policies for reducing substance abuse. Perhaps more important, it nurtured researchers who had turned their attention to substance abuse. "It cut across a lot of different fields, bringing in economists, political scientists, sociologists, public health experts, legal researchers, and others," said Frank Chaloupka, director of the Health Policy Center at the University of Illinois Chicago and a frequent SAPRP grantee. "It provided support for work that never would have been done otherwise. Substance abuse policy research involved a very small group at the beginning, but SAPRP brought many new people into the field."

Results from SAPRP-funded grants assist policymakers, government administrators, judicial systems, the media, advocacy groups, community organizations, and private organizations such as HMOs, employers, associations, and trade groups in making informed decisions on substance abuse issues. To date, SAPRP has funded more than 360 projects. SAPRP-funded research has been published in major peer-reviewed journals, featured in national and local media, and included in testimony before Congress, state legislatures, and city councils.

Bridging the Gap

In 1997, the Foundation established Bridging the Gap, a $57.2 million research initiative that sought to expand understanding about the impact of policies, programs, and environmental factors on the health behaviors—and substance abuse choices—of adolescents. The most recent re-authorization, in October 2008, continues the program through 2012, but with a changed orientation, primarily focusing on the determinants of childhood obesity and secondarily on smoking by young people.

An important part of Bridging the Gap's work during the first authorization (1997–2006) was based on the annual Monitoring the Future (MTF) surveys. Funded by NIDA, MTF has been conducting school-based surveys of high school seniors since 1975 and eighth-grade and tenth-grade students since 1991. About 50,000 adolescents in 420 schools nationwide are surveyed each spring. The data collected encompass substance use, attitudes, and beliefs about substance use, availability of various substances, exposure to anti-drug advertising, and more.

Using MTF data, Bridging the Gap had two integrated components: Youth, Education, and Society (YES), based at the University of Michigan's Institute for Social Research, and ImpacTeen, based at the Health Policy Center at the University of Illinois at Chicago. The YES project surveyed school administrators annually about alcohol, tobacco, and illicit drug-related policies and how they are implemented. The survey also collected information on prevention and cessation programs and curriculums. ImpacTeen gathered a range of data at the state and community levels on such issues as illicit drug-related ordinances, anti-illicit drug advertising, activities to address youth substance abuse, and after-school programs.

These databases were mined to improve understanding of how policies, programs, and other factors influence adolescent substance use and abuse. Some analyses raised questions about whether school drug testing has a significant effect on student drug use. Others have shown that marijuana use among youth decreases as marijuana prices and perceived harmfulness rise.

National Center on Addiction and Substance Abuse

Founded in 1992 by Joseph Califano, Jr., a former US secretary of health, education, and welfare, The National Center on

Addiction and Substance Abuse at Columbia University (CASA) aims to inform Americans about the economic and social costs of substance abuse and its impact on their lives, and strives to remove the stigma of substance abuse. When CASA arrived on the scene, according to Califano, the field lacked a comprehensive approach to substance abuse: "There was no model. There was no place in the country that [said] the problem is addiction and not one related to any particular substance. Whether it's nicotine, alcohol, pills, drugs, illegal drugs, or steroids, the issue is addiction and abuse. Number two, the concept was that you'd get all different disciplines, not just medicine and law, but sociology, anthropology, statistics, communications, business, labor to look at abuse of all substances, in all parts of society, not just the health care system and the criminal justice system but also the impact on the family, schools, child welfare, the welfare system, the homeless, on property and vandalism, and on productivity. That was the concept. It was the one place where you brought together all the skills to look at all substance abuse in all parts of society."

The Robert Wood Johnson Foundation has provided $56 million to CASA. With a staff of more than sixty professionals with postgraduate and doctoral degrees, CASA produces several major reports every year. In 2007, the reports covered binge drinking and abuse of prescription and illegal drugs on college campuses, prescription drug pushers on the Internet, an annual teen survey on substance abuse, and white papers on the importance of family dinners in deterring drug, alcohol, and tobacco use.

CASA has launched several projects that seek to convert its research findings into institutional change in four areas: working with families to help them recognize teen substance abuse; reducing illegal drug use among girls and young women; developing a bill of rights for juvenile offenders; and calling on the Food and Drug Administration to issue new rules requiring pharmaceutical companies to formulate drugs that minimize the potential for intentional and unintentional abuse.

To Califano, one of CASA's signal policy successes came with the advent of drug courts, where offenders can have their indictments and convictions expunged if they successfully follow a counseling and treatment regimen. "We did an analysis of the first three drug courts that found that they were effective in reducing recidivism," Califano said. "It led to the federal support of drug courts, and today there are 2,000 around the country. But the number one thing we've done is finding that it's all about getting a kid through age twenty-one without smoking, without using illegal drugs, and without abusing alcohol. If we can, that kid is virtually certain to be home free. And the parents have the greatest influence on their children, for better or worse."

CASA's combination of research and advocacy—along with controversy over the accuracy and reliability of its research—has produced some mixed reviews. *The Chronicle of Higher Education* once noted that Califano "has won plaudits for taking on not only shadowy drug kingpins, but also alcohol companies and Big Tobacco," but also that "CASA has also been accused of playing fast and loose with statistics, skirting the academic peer-review process in favor of grandstanding, and acting as an unskeptical cheerleader for the war on drugs."[2] In 2009, CASA merged with Join Together, a Boston-based substance abuse research and advocacy organization, that also has been funded by the Robert Wood Johnson Foundation.

Developing Leadership in Reducing Substance Abuse and Innovators Combating Substance Abuse

In the early 1990s, when Foundation staff members looked for leading researchers to serve on advisory committees, review grant proposals, and undertake other activities to inform the Foundation's grant making, they could identify only a small group of people. To remedy this, the Foundation decided to develop a cadre of new substance abuse research leaders, including those from varied racial, ethnic, and professional groups and coming from fields such as public policy, public health, and journalism.[3] In 2000, it announced two new programs: Developing Leadership in Reducing Substance Abuse, aimed at nurturing a new generation of research leaders in the substance abuse field, and Innovators Combating Substance Abuse, that would recognize established researchers and their contributions.

Developing Leadership offered three-year fellowships to ten individuals a year who showed promise as leaders in research on substance abuse prevention, treatment, and policy. The program also featured a mentoring component to attract more minority scholars, and scheduled regular meetings to support the fellows. The program selected forty fellows in total. When it closed in 2006, Judith Schector, the national program director, said. "The overall results are forty people who were able to significantly advance their careers. It's too soon to know the impact. It's hard to imagine that these forty people over time will not have an impact on the field."[4]

Innovators Combating Substance Abuse provided five awards a year to senior researchers. Twenty researchers received awards between 2000 and 2003. In late 2007, the national program office published a book, *Addiction Treatment: Science and Policy for the 21ˢᵗ Century,* which featured more than two dozen essays by innovation award-winners.[5]

—⨲— Strategies to Counter Drug Abuse at the Community Level

During the 1990s and early 2000s, the Foundation experimented with a range of models to combat substance abuse, including drug abuse. One was the formation of community coalitions, a concept that emerged from the War on Poverty in the 1960s and had become popular among philanthropies in the 1980s as a way of encouraging bottom-up solutions to social problems. The coalitions brought together a broad band of community groups and citizens in the hope of developing coordinated strategies to prevent the spread of drug abuse. The Foundation also worked to prevent young people ensnared in the criminal justice system from returning to drugs by improving the way judges, probation officers, treatment providers, families, and community members approach the problem of juveniles and substance abuse.

Fighting Back: Community Initiatives to Reduce Demand for Illegal Drugs and Alcohol

The surge in the use of crack cocaine in the mid-1980s spurred the Foundation to undertake one of its earliest efforts at combating drug (and also alcohol) abuse, Fighting Back. Launched in 1988, the theory behind Fighting Back was to establish community coalitions composed of a broad range of citizens, agencies, and organizations that would work together in combating substance abuse.[6] Fighting Back was, in effect, a test of the theory that broad-based community coalitions could have a real impact on reducing substance abuse, and the Foundation mandated a rigid framework that required a citizens' task force on drug and alcohol abuse—a communitywide consortium of the institutions, organizations, and agencies whose participation would be needed to implement the program.

In 1998, the Foundation transferred Fighting Back's national program office from Vanderbilt University to Join Together, another Foundation-supported organization, at the Boston University School of Public Health. Also at that time, the Foundation ended funding to six of the original fourteen communities participating in the program. David Rosenbloom, director of Join Together, changed both the governance structure—dropping the required structure of citizens' task forces—and the direction of the program, to emphasize the development of services to treat and deter substance abuse.

In 2003, a team of evaluators at Brandeis University delivered a report that found no significant decrease in substance abuse in Fighting Back sites when compared with demographically similar communities. Advocates for the program contested the results, pointing out flaws in the methodology, the survey sample, and the funding. They emphasized that the evaluation, which began after the program was well under way, did not have a reliable baseline against which to measure.

James Knickman, formerly the Foundation's vice president for research and evaluation, rejected the criticisms and noted that for an investment of nearly $70 million the Foundation had every right to expect more tangible results.[7] "The bottom line," he said in an interview for a Foundation Grant Results Report, "is that the results indicate that the Fighting Back approach does not offer a solution to the substance abuse problem."[8]

Join Together and Community Anti-Drug Coalitions of America

Even as Fighting Back was getting up and running, the federal government adopted the model and funded 251 community anti-substance-abuse coalitions under the Drug-Free Communities Act. This surge in the number of coalitions led the Foundation to fund two organizations—Join Together in 1991 and Community Anti-Drug Coalitions of America, or CADCA, in 1992—to nurture the coalitions and provide them with technical support. Join Together and CADCA offered substantially different approaches to technical support. CADCA is a membership organization that, in addition to providing technical assistance, acts as a trade organization in Washington, D.C. Join Together has a policy analysis and publication agenda and maintains a highly regarded Web site that directs readers to a large array of resources related to substance abuse.

In addition to its online service, Join Together produces and sends out newsletters, reports, and monthly action kits to its large mailing list, helping readers keep abreast of relevant trends and issues and offering guidance on specific actions that local leaders could take to address those issues in their communities.

The program also established the Join Together Fellows program. During one-year fellowships, fellows are brought together three times for sessions on leadership development, strategic planning, and other content areas, such as advances in prevention research and updates on new public policy developments in the field. In 2009, Join Together merged into CASA, and David Rosenbloom was named CASA president and CEO.

Free to Grow: Head Start Partnerships to Promote Substance-Free Communities

In the early 1990s, the Foundation developed a wide-ranging anti-drug-and-alcohol experiment launched in partnership with the federal Head Start preschool program. Called Free to Grow, it was authorized in 1992 for testing in six communities and expanded in 2000 to fifteen sites.[9] The program closed in April 2007.

Free to Grow provided no direct services to Head Start youngsters. Instead, it brought together broad-based community partners in efforts to strengthen families and communities to address a young child's overall environment. The program was based on a body of research that identified family and neighborhood characteristics that can heighten or moderate the risk of substance abuse and other harmful activities. Using the structural framework of Head Start to reach needy families and neighborhoods, Free to Grow fostered partnerships among existing community and family service organizations, police, and government agencies to mitigate the threats to children.

The program defined threat broadly. Obvious threats—addicted or abusive family members and roving street gangs—shared attention with subtler threats, such as vermin-infested housing, lack of supervised after-school programs, and hostility between neighborhood residents and police. Many of Free to Grow's activities were only tangentially related to substance abuse; the program included initiatives against crime, negligent landlords, unemployment, adult illiteracy, language barriers, and even traffic problems.

The sites came up with various strategies to strengthen families and communities, including assessment and case management, referral to counseling and treatment, parent education classes, peer mentoring, and support groups. Strategies to strengthen communities included organizing residents and existing groups to survey neighborhood needs, working together on solutions, building leadership skills, and fostering partnerships among existing local agencies. Across sites, two partners jumped out from the pilot phase as critically important: schools and police. Schools weren't surprising, because they shared Head Start's education mission. But the interest and the enthusiasm of police were unexpected. As the program played out, police would surpass local educators as Free to Grow's strongest allies and advocates.

Free to Grow benefited more from broader public support for safeguarding innocent young people than from support aimed at helping already troubled teenagers or adults escape the consequences of bad choices. In this context, Free to Grow's environmental interventions—like better housing code enforcement, neighborhood cleanup, traffic safety, and supervised after-school programs—were easy sells. But the program's long-term goal—less drinking and drug taking—remained elusive.[10]

—∿— Young People in the Criminal Justice System—Reclaiming Futures: Communities Helping Teens Overcome Drugs, Alcohol, and Crime

Research shows that young people who abuse drugs and alcohol are more likely to behave violently or to end up in court. As many as four in five teens in trouble with the law are abusing drugs and alcohol.[11] But substance abuse treatment in the juvenile court system is often haphazard, ineffective, or nonexistent. Without proper treatment, many young people fall back into a life that gets them into trouble with the law. By funding the Reclaiming Futures program, the Foundation sought to test ways to make widespread improvements in how the juvenile justice system handles young people with drug problems.[12]

Started in 2002, Reclaiming Futures created and evaluated a new approach to help teens caught in the cycle of substance abuse and crime. It was implemented in ten cities nationwide and sought to improve the way judges, probation officers, treatment providers, families, and community members approached the problem of juveniles and substance abuse. The initiative was community focused and emphasized cooperation among a range of agencies and groups—courts, service providers, community organizations, schools, health organizations, and individual volunteers—to meet the needs of young people in the juvenile justice system. The model required juvenile justice and treatment systems to work together across agency boundaries and increase their involvement with the community at large.

The Urban Institute and Chapin Hall at the University of Chicago published an evaluation of Reclaiming Futures in 2006. It found that across the ten project communities, twelve of the thirteen indicators of coordination between the juvenile justice and substance abuse treatment centers showed significant improvements. At the same time, the evaluators pointed out that it was premature to evaluate whether the program had led to improved outcomes among the individuals that it served.

In 2007 and 2008, The Robert Wood Johnson Foundation, two federal government agencies, and one other foundation expanded Reclaiming Futures to sixteen new communities. The Robert Wood Johnson Foundation's funds are being used to support the national program office at Portland State University.

—⚏— Communications and the Media—The Partnership for a Drug-Free America

Staff members at the Foundation realized that there were many substance abuse issues that would be well beyond the reach of the organizations it funded that were working at the local level. "We knew that there had to be some programs operating at the national level," recalled Paul Jellinek, a former Foundation vice president. "The coalitions did not have enough leverage on this issue on their own."

Jellinek was working with the then-Foundation senior vice president Ruby Hearn to devise such national programs. But the impetus to broaden the reach of the Foundation's substance abuse programming came not from the staff but from one of the Foundation's trustees, James Burke, the former CEO of Johnson & Johnson who is probably best known for his crisis management in 1982, when Tylenol capsules were found to be poisoned with cyanide. Burke had served as chairman of the Partnership for a Drug-Free America, a private, nonprofit coalition of professionals from the communications industry that had been creating pro bono national media-based anti-drug (and other substances) campaigns since 1986. "Burke believed," Jellinek said, "that the way to go was to mobilize all this marketing and advertising talent to 'unsell' drugs."

"We got a proposal from the Partnership, Ruby Hearn and I reviewed it, and, without taking Jim Burke into consideration, we thought it made a lot of sense," Jellinek said. Between 1989 and 2009, the Foundation supported the Partnership with grants totaling nearly $56 million. Over the course of the grants, the Partnership secured more than $2.3 billion in donated advertising time and space and developed more than 1,000 public service announcements for print, television, and radio outlets.[13]

The Partnership's goal is to reduce adolescents' demand for illicit drugs by warning them about the hazards (perhaps its most memorable ad was the 1987 "This is your brain on drugs" print and TV ad, which featured a frying pan and a fried egg) and by equipping parents with the skills to communicate effectively with their children about the perils of drug and alcohol abuse. Its annual survey, the Partnership Attitude Tracking Study, monitors consumer attitudes about illicit drugs, which in turn helps shape media campaigns and hones the tools that the Partnership offers to parents in counseling their children. A Web site offers toolkits for parents, information aimed at teens, treatment help for drug abusers, and detailed information on many types of illicit drugs.

The Partnership's most recent annual survey, released in February 2009, showed the first major increase in the number of teens who reported "learning a lot" about the risks of drugs from their parents. The study shows that 37 percent of teens reported learning a lot about the risks of drugs from their parents, a 16 percent increase from the previous year and the first major increase since the inception of the study.[14] The study also indicated a strong correlation between increased teen exposure to anti-drug messages on television and a decreased likelihood of trying drugs over the past ten years.

"The Partnership is the premier communications organization in the addiction field," Thomas McLellan, the co-founder and chief executive officer of the Treatment Research Institute in Philadelphia until his recent appointment as deputy director of the federal Office of National Drug Control Policy, said. "It has unique capacities to distill the important scientific findings and to reach literally millions of parents and other consumers through their media connections." Added former Foundation vice president Jellinek, "Inherently, there's real value in having these ads run on TV saying that [drugs] are not all right, that they're dangerous. That message is out there in the national bloodstream. But I think it's very hard to know how effective any of the Partnership's efforts have been."

—ᴑᴑ— Improving the Treatment Process

Drug addiction—a sprawling, messy, complex social and health problem—defies a unified approach. Over recent decades, those in the prevention camp have vied for funding with those in the treatment camp, while researchers have embarked on thousands of projects in efforts to establish an ever-growing canon of evidence-based data and practices. Just as patterns of drug abuse have changed over the years, with crack cocaine surging in the 1980s and abuse of prescription drugs mounting today, the approaches to prevention and treatment have evolved as well.

Starting in the mid-1990s, scientific advances in brain research were solidifying support for the proposition that addiction is a brain disease that develops over time as a result of initially voluntary behavior of using drugs. Addiction, researchers said, comes about through an array of neurological changes. The evidence suggests that long-lasting brain changes are responsible for the distortions of cognitive and emotional functioning that are the essence of addiction.[15] Against this backdrop, in the late 1990s growing numbers of researchers and experts came to view addiction as a chronic health condition. At the Foundation, the perception of addiction as a chronic health condition was also taking hold.

Enter Victor Capoccia, who had been recruited to the Foundation in 2001 and whose clinical experience and doctoral studies had led him to conclude that addiction is really a chronic illness. When he joined the Foundation, the relevant team within the Foundation was named Alcohol and Illegal Drugs. "That's looking at it as a social issue," said Capoccia. "We didn't have a team called the fatty foods team; we didn't have team called the deadly tobacco team. But we had the Alcohol and Illegal Drugs team, and, symbolically, you're attaching stigma. That's not what you should do with a health condition." The name morphed into the Addiction Prevention and Treatment Team to reflect the field's growing commitment to viewing addiction as a chronic illness, and the Foundation developed a trio of programs—Paths to Recovery, Resources for Recovery, and Advancing Recovery—aimed at improving the quality of treatment.

Paths to Recovery: Changing the Process of Care for Substance Abuse

At any given time, more than 20 million Americans need substance abuse treatment, but fewer than 10 percent get appointments for treatment. Of this 10 percent, fewer than half show up for their appointments.[16] The Foundation's new Addiction Prevention and Treatment Team sought to make dramatic improvements in those numbers by increasing access to drug and alcohol treatment, improving the quality of treatment, and strengthening the nation's addiction treatment infrastructure.

In seeking to narrow the gulf between needed substance abuse treatments and burdensome processes that get in the way, the Foundation established Paths to Recovery, which selected ten sites nationwide to participate in a "learning collaborative" to identify and share the best treatment practices. In 2005, the Foundation funded thirteen more sites and the federal Center for Substance Abuse Treatment added another thirteen. To create a system that was less frustrating for both clients and staff and would make it easier to complete treatment, the sites made changes, based on business models, in client intake procedures, assessment, scheduling, outreach, and family involvement.

"Common in drug and alcohol treatment programs are long delays between the time a person calls a program for treatment and the time that appointment is available, and as a result 50 percent of the people who are scheduled for appointments don't show up," said Dennis McCarty, a professor in the Department of Public Health and Preventive Medicine at Oregon Health and Science University and the evaluator of the Paths to Recovery and Advancing Recovery programs. "That's inefficient for the program and inconvenient for the client."

The mechanism that was set up for sharing information about best practices is called the Network for the Improvement of Addiction Treatment (NIATx), housed at the University of Wisconsin-Madison and directed by David Gustafson, emeritus professor of engineering. A partnership among Paths to Recovery, the Strengthening Treatment Access and Retention (STAR) program of the Center for Substance Abuse Treatment, and a number of independent addiction treatment organizations, NIATx offers learning opportunities and technical support to alcohol and drug treatment centers in four problem areas: reducing waiting times, reducing no-shows, increasing admissions, and increasing continuation of treatment. "Participating treatment programs get coaching from experts experienced in business process improvement," said McCarty. "The focus is on doing one thing at a time, don't make it too complicated, don't plan forever, and just take an action."

NIATx offers site visits by its staff members, and further technical support is available through its Web site, conference calls on specific topics, and video-conferencing. Since its inception, NIATx has provided technical support to nearly 1,000 treatment agencies.[17] According to the NIATx Web site, participating programs over the past four years have realized improvements in all of its focus areas: 34 percent reduction in waiting times, 33 percent reduction in no-shows, 21 percent increase in admissions, and 22 percent increase in treatment continuation.[18]

"NIATx has had a tremendous impact on the field," McCarty said. "These programs made changes in how they delivered care, got people into care quicker, and kept them in care longer. And many of the programs increased the numbers of admissions, reduced their no-shows, and reduced their costs so that they were more efficient and were generating more income than at the start of the project." SAMHSA's Jack Stein agreed. "There was a level of innovation that allowed us to think outside the box. . . .

Applying business practices to the community-based substance abuse treatment field [was] a major shift in how we do business."

Resources for Recovery: State Practices that Expand Treatment Opportunities

Resources for Recovery was designed to improve linkages between state drug and alcohol treatment agencies and state Medicaid agencies, with the idea of expanding treatment capacity and people served. It provided funds for experts in state financing to help states maximize the potential benefits from major federal programs targeting addiction prevention and treatment.[19]

The program took place in fifteen states. "In many states, those relationships were not well developed," McCarty said. "Resources for Recovery provided coaching, consultation, and technical assistance to help states revise their Medicaid plans so that those plans would include treatment for drug and alcohol disorders. The idea was to improve financing for drug abuse treatment so we can get more people into care."

But, according to Thomas McLellan, the former CEO of the Treatment Research Institute in Philadelphia who is currently the deputy director of the federal Office of National Drug Control Policy, "It is fair to say that over the years in drug abuse treatment, states have lost interest, lost hope, reduced their budgets, and made more use of federal dollars. In these bad budgetary times, no one is eager to take on new programs. So these state systems are really not conducive to implementing some of the potential advances."

Advancing Recovery: State/Provider Partnerships for Quality Addiction Care

Advancing Recovery is a collaboration among the Robert Wood Johnson Foundation, NIATx, the Treatment Research Institute, and six payer-provider partnerships, chosen in two rounds (six two-year awards were made in 2006 and another six in 2008).

It promotes the use of evidence-based clinical practices through partnerships between state agencies and substance abuse treatment organizations and builds on the work of NIATx by improving the potential for sustained change in treatment system financing, regulation, and purchasing.

"Advancing Recovery applies the NIATx concept—let's improve our treatment processes and system—and looks at the linkages between the state agency that's funding these services and the treatment programs themselves," McCarty said. "So if you want to use medication to improve treatment for drug and alcohol disorders, you need to make sure you've got payment systems in place for the medication. You need to make sure you have regulations set up so that treatment programs can use the medication."

McLellan, the program's former co-director (Gustafson, the national program director of NIATx at the University of Wisconsin–Madison, is the other co-director), said Advancing Recovery's combination of implementing effective practices at the program level with effective purchasing, organization, and financing practices at the state level makes sense. "Around 75 percent of all addiction treatment episodes are funded by states," he said. "This is an area that the private sector has basically walked away from. So it was a great idea, but I think it has been only a partial success. The NIATx component continues to be excellent, but it would be charitable to say that the states have been 50 percent effective in getting to understand and be able to correct fundamental problems in how they manage treatment systems."

—〜— The Retreat from Addiction Prevention and Treatment

In 2006, the Foundation announced its decision that it would not continue to make addiction prevention and treatment a priority. Foundation President and CEO Risa Lavizzo-Mourey explained the rationale for the decision. "I think the work in prevention had led to organizations that were established and mature and were able to continue on because they had been long-term players in the field," she said. "And the areas that were relatively new—quality of treatment—were so new that we realized we were certainly at a crossroads. We either had to stay there for a long time, giving them enough to take the lessons that they've learned and run with them, or begin an exit. So I think the decision was borne out of an understanding of what it would take to continue in an area, treatment, where we really didn't have the resources to do everything we wanted, and seeing that, on the prevention side, we had organizations that were pretty mature. Although I'm not diminishing how tough it would be, they were certainly at a point where it was possible and very probable, even if difficult, to continue without our support."

To long-time grantees, fellow advocates, and partners, the Foundation's decision to step away from the drug addiction field was met with dismay, leavened by grudging doses of reality. "There is concern among investigators in the field that the absence of Robert Wood Johnson Foundation funding will impede progress, particularly in policy research," said David Altman, the director of the Substance Abuse Policy and Research Program. "That said, it's unusual for a foundation to be invested in a field for so long, so I can understand why they are redirecting their investments to other pressing public health matters." Because it had been such a large presence in the field—so large that it acted as a disincentive for other funders to join in—the Foundation's departure left a gaping hole in the drug addiction arena. "At its peak, the Robert Wood Johnson Foundation was putting more than $70 million a year into services and research. You can't lose $70 million and not have a negative impact." said Oregon Health and Science University Professor McCarty.

"Whenever you announce you're winding down or leaving a field that you helped create, have supported substantially for a long time, and whose practitioners are so passionate about, it's going to cause angst, pushback, and even some antagonism," David Morse, vice president for communications at the Foundation, said. "But we have wound down slowly, and I hope responsibly, to cause as little disruption as possible, and we are capturing and sharing the learning and lessons we've gleaned from twenty-plus years of investment in the addiction field, to strengthen the base we've helped build."

—᠁— The Foundation's Impact on the Field of Drug Addiction

Before its decision to leave the field in 2006, the Robert Wood Johnson Foundation had, for more than twenty years, played a significant role in the field of drug addiction. As part of its exit strategy, the Foundation, in 2007, commissioned Laufer Green Isaac, a marketing communications firm based Los Angeles, to conduct a survey of current and former leaders of the Robert Wood Johnson Foundation and other foundations, current and former grantees, other foundations, and leaders in the field in order to gain a better understanding of the Foundation's legacy in the addiction prevention and treatment field, including tobacco.

The survey found that the Foundation's role was generally not well known outside of the community with which it interacted. "Among other funders we interviewed, there was low awareness and knowledge of the Foundation's work in addiction," said Jessica Laufer, the CEO of Laufer Green Isaac. "The interviewees couldn't describe it. Only those in direct contact with staff or grantees said the Foundation was considered an addiction prevention and treatment leader in the philanthropic community. Those without direct proximity to the Foundation didn't see it in that way."

Despite uneven recognition of its drug addiction work, however, the Foundation had amassed, in the eyes of the survey group, substantial achievements. The survey report lists three in particular:

- Its role in building the national infrastructure for the field, including a significant contribution to building community coalitions

- Its role in funding policy research
- Its willingness to fund innovative and risky projects

Former program officers, government researchers, grantees, and a former Foundation president were asked for their own, on-the-record, observations, looking back at what the Foundation accomplished and where it could have done better. What emerges is a consensus: That the Foundation played a key role, especially through the Substance Abuse Policy Research Program, in funding the research that became the bedrock of policy formation; that its drug prevention demonstration projects in community coalitions had uneven success, despite the widespread adoption of the model nationally; that several programs, namely CADCA, Join Together, and CASA, were successful and lasting contributors to the field (although the Laufer Green Isaac findings noted that CASA was just as likely to be cited negatively for its controversial research techniques); and that its late-blooming focus on improving the treatment process yielded the effective and much praised NIATx learning collaborative.

On balance, then, the Foundation's sizable investment in addiction prevention and treatment was considered a qualified success, weakened by a lack of a strong, steady strategic vision, episodic program decisions, and some institutional infighting. And looming constantly over the fragmented drug addiction work was the Foundation's signature accomplishment: its highly regarded efforts to reduce smoking. It proved to be a very tough act to follow.

For Steven Schroeder, who presided over the growth of the Foundation's substance abuse work in the 1990s, it was the federal government's engagement in the drug abuse field in the 1980s—combined with the Foundation's entry into the arena—that had the broadest effect. "Whether that was because of us, in spite of us, or we were riding a wave that was out of our control, it's hard to say," Schroeder recalled. "The general sense we had was that it was hard to tell that our individual programs made a lot of difference. But it's unquestionable that the country is in a much better place now with regard to drug abuse, especially cocaine, than when these programs got started. A lot of people think that the Foundation's getting out there early helped to get the federal government involved. We helped to galvanize a movement [but] whether any of our specific models can be seen as 'ah ha' models isn't as clear to me."

The Foundation's decision to shift the emphasis from prevention to treatment and the adoption of a team approach to making decisions about grants created its own in-house problems. "It was a difficult priority because you had a lot of programs ongoing that were traditional prevention programs," said Constance Pechura, a former senior program officer in the drug addiction area and currently the executive director of the Treatment Research Institute. "So there was a challenge of doing new programs with somewhat limited funds on top of old legacy programs."

Many people consider the lack of a long-term strategic framework to have blunted the impact of the Foundation's drug addiction work. The assault on tobacco deployed a four-pronged attack: policy research; state-level advocacy; a nimble national communications and advocacy office (the Campaign for Tobacco-Free Kids); and prevention and cessation programs tightly focused on a single drug, nicotine. Largely untethered and without an aggressive advocacy voice like the Campaign for Tobacco-Free Kids, the Foundation's drug addiction work never settled into a coordinated scheme. Unlike the tobacco strategy, which started off much the same way but coalesced into a highly effective model, the drug addiction work was more scattershot, "up to the whims of whoever was running it at the time," as one Foundation program officer put it.

And the field itself—disparate and asymmetrical—proved to be much more daunting than tobacco. "The Robert Wood Johnson Foundation effort addressed very important problem areas in the substance abuse service system, but the system they were attempting to influence is very complex and confusing," said Rick Rawson, a professor in the Department of Psychiatry at UCLA with decades of expertise in the substance abuse arena. "The audience it was trying to influence was too diverse and heterogeneous," Rawson continued. "That wasn't so true with cigarettes."

To Jessica Laufer, the comparison between the Foundation's work to reduce smoking and to reduce drug abuse is not a fair one. "Clearly, tobacco was a much hotter issue," Laufer said. "There was a big lawsuit and it had much more visibility. But I don't think you can say the Foundation's work in tobacco outweighs that in the drug addiction area. It's a little bit like comparing apples and oranges, because the emphasis was much more on a public platform with tobacco. The Foundation proactively and heavily communicated its involvement in tobacco, but not so much in the addiction area, so there was overall a lack of awareness of the addiction prevention and treatment work."

David Altman, the director of the Substance Abuse Policy Research Program, noted that the Robert Wood Foundation had funded tobacco policy research longer than it had funded drug policy research. "Their funding of tobacco demonstration projects and advocacy and education organizations was more robust than in the drug area," Altman wrote in an e-mail. "Also, the context of tobacco and drugs is very different. One big issue is that in tobacco there are centralized tobacco companies (or a tobacco industry), whereas in the drug area, control and influence are more decentralized. Finally, the policy options are different. Nicotine policies include taxes, access, marketing, and treatment. Policies on drugs (including abuse of prescription drugs) relate more to treatment and impact on publicly funded services, such as housing, welfare, and treatment."

"The policy levers available for tobacco control were much better defined and much easier to exercise," McCarty, of Oregon Health and Science University, said. "Excise taxes, second-hand smoke—these were pieces of the puzzle that tobacco folks picked up on and were able manipulate and tweak." In addition, while public attitudes toward smoking have hardened dramatically, attitudes toward drug use remain more nuanced. "The nation has been much more ambivalent about drug use and whether it's been good or bad," McCarty said. "The ongoing debate over marijuana as medicine is evidence of that ambivalence. I think drug addiction is a more complex set of behaviors, disorders, and problems."

"Did it accomplish all it intended to do? No, but it's always hard to know what would have happened in the absence of those efforts," said Joan Hollendonner, a former senior communications officer at the Foundation who oversaw many of its substance abuse programs. "I think for learning and experimenting, it gets an 'A.' Community coalitions and some of these other approaches weren't tried and true. It was a bit of pioneering. Were some differences made? Yes. Was the problem solved? No. So I think it's a mixed bag. Compared with tobacco, it hasn't made as much progress."

Given the thorny problems inherent in combating drug abuse—social, health, political, scientific, moral—it is little wonder that the Foundation's legacy is ambiguous. "I don't think we will be able to know for some years to come what our impact has been," Lavizzo-Mourey said. "There have been a lot of leaders in the field who got their start as a result of Robert Wood Johnson Foundation funding and other kinds of support. I think the long-term impact of the work that was funded over fifteen to twenty years will ultimately speak for itself . . . because there is a lot of good work by a lot of good people, and we will see how that turns out."

Notes

1. Gutman, M. A., Altman, D. G., and Rabin, R. L. "Tobacco Policy Research." *To Improve Health and Health Care: The Robert Wood Johnson Foundation Anthology, 1998–1999.* San Francisco: Jossey-Bass, 1999.
2. Shea, C. "In Drug-Policy Debates, a Center at Columbia U. Takes a Hard Line." *The Chronicle of Higher Education,* October 3, 1997.
3. Robert Wood Johnson Foundation. "Creating Leadership Development in Reducing Substance Abuse." *Grant Results Report,* February 2008.

http://www.rwjf.org/reports/npreports/devleader.htm. Accessed on June 6, 2009.

4. Ibid.

5. Robert Wood Johnson Foundation. "Addiction Treatment: Science and Policy for the Twenty-First Century Selected as Outstanding Academic Title." *Grant Results Report*, February 12, 2009. http://www.rwjf.org/pr/product.jsp?id=38808. Accessed on June 6, 2009.

6. See Wielawski, I. "The Fighting Back Program." *To Improve Health and Health Care: The Robert Wood Johnson Foundation Anthology, Vol. VII*. San Francisco: Jossey-Bass, 2004.

7. Knickman, J. R. "Fighting Back: A Funder's Perspective." *Journal of Drug Issues*, 36, 2006, 467–482.

8. Robert Wood Johnson Foundation. "Fighting Back." *Grant Results Report*, 2007. http://www.rwjf.org/pr/product.jsp?id=16956. Accessed on June 6, 2009.

9. Wielawski, I. "Free to Grow." *To Improve Health and Health Care: The Robert Wood Johnson Foundation Anthology, Vol. IX*. San Francisco: Jossey-Bass, 2006.

10. Ibid.

11. Binard, J., and Prichard, M. *Model Policies for Juvenile Justice and Substance Abuse Treatment: A Report by Reclaiming Futures*. The Robert Wood Johnson Foundation, 2008.

12. See Solovitch, S., "Reclaiming Futures," chapter 7 of this *Anthology*, for a fuller discussion of the program.

13. Robert Wood Johnson Foundation. "Madison Avenue Sells a Strong New Message: Drugs Aren't Cool." *Grant Results Report*, January 2001. http://www.rwjf.org/reports/grr/022753s.htm. Accessed on June 6, 2009.

14. The Partnership for a Drug-Free America. *20th Annual Teen Study Shows 25 Percent Drop in Meth Use over Three Years; Marijuana Down 30 Percent over Ten Years*, April 20, 2009. http://www.drugfree.org/Portal/About/NewsReleases/20th_Annual_Teen_Study. Accessed on June 8, 2009.

15. Leshner, A. I. "Addiction Is a Brain Disease." *Issues in Science and Technology*, spring 2001. http://www.issues.org/17.3/leshner.htm. Accessed on June 6, 2009.

16. "NIATx Overview." https://www.niatx.net/Content/ContentPage.aspx?NID=9. Accessed on June 8, 2009.

17. Ibid.

18. Ibid.

19. Robert Wood Johnson Foundation. "Resources for Recovery: State Practices that Expand Treatment Resources Recovery." *Grant Results Report*, July 27, 2007. www.rwjf.org/pr/product.jsp?id=19651. Accessed on June 8, 2009.

Reclaiming Futures

Sara Solovitch

In her freshman year of high school, Courtney J., an Anchorage teenager with all-American looks honed by years of swimming laps and flying down mountain faces on her skis, started drinking and smoking marijuana—a drug she took to so quickly that, as she remembers telling herself after the third time, she intended to do it every day for the rest of her life. By the time summer came, she had lost all her friends on the swim team and was dropping Ecstasy and cocaine every weekend. In her sophomore year, she began experimenting with methamphetamine; over the next eight months, she missed forty-five days of school and failed two classes. She missed her junior year altogether.

Her mother, Carolyn, searched the Internet and called providers in the Lower 48 states, but quickly concluded that the only way to make her daughter enter treatment would be to have her arrested. Once, when she had tried driving her to a residential treatment facility, Courtney jumped out of the car while it was moving at twenty-five miles an hour. Convinced that the answer lay in the juvenile justice system, Carolyn bided her time and waited "for one of those little openings."

Over the previous three years, Courtney had been picked up for shoplifting, drinking, and assault (she had stabbed a friend's hand while in a drunken fit). She had spent two weeks in the McLaughlin Youth Center, a secure state-run detention facility on thirteen acres across the street from the University of Alaska in Anchorage, and six months at the Adolescent Residential Center for Help, a treatment program for chemically dependent youth in nearby Eagle River.

The latest "little opening," the one that got her into her third round of treatment, came in December 2007 as Courtney, then eighteen, was leaving the house at two in the morning. When Carolyn forbade her to walk out the door, Courtney hit her mother in the ear. It wasn't really so bad, Carolyn says now, sneaking a rueful look at her daughter. But it was the excuse she needed. She called the police, and Courtney was once again processed through the juvenile justice system—this time as a client of Reclaiming Futures, an initiative of the Robert Wood Johnson Foundation then in its fifth and final year.

—∿— The Development of Reclaiming Futures

As Courtney's mother had discovered several years ago, few treatment resources exist for teenagers and adolescents outside the criminal justice system. Nationally, fewer than one in ten young people with drug and alcohol problems get any treatment, according to the federal Substance Abuse and Mental Health Services Administration (SAMHSA), and of the estimated 150,000 that do, less than 25 percent stay in treatment for three months—the minimum time recommended by the National Institute on Drug Abuse. According to SAMHSA, fewer than 50 percent stay for even six weeks.[1]

Inside the system, it isn't much better. Despite research showing that treating alcohol and drug abuse reduces crime, the vast majority of incarcerated young people receive no treatment at all. Nevertheless, the situation is much improved from a decade ago, when rigorous evidence-based treatment programs for adolescents were almost nonexistent. Prior to 1997, a total of fourteen studies had been published in the field of adolescent drug treatment, and many of those were widely regarded as being of questionable quality. All that began changing in the last decade—around the same time program officers at the Robert Wood Johnson Foundation started laying the groundwork for Reclaiming Futures. Although more is now known about treating adolescents who are addicted, a basic lack of knowledge continues to this day, especially about why substance use turns into addiction in some young people and not others. According to the National Institute on Alcohol Abuse and Alcoholism, many young people appear to simply "age out" of substance abuse.[2] The challenge is in trying to identify which will fall into the other half and move on to a lifetime of chronic addiction.

Over the past decade, the field has exploded with dozens of new federal grants, hundreds of studies, new interventions, and evaluations of program outcomes. One of the interventions was Reclaiming Futures, a $30 million initiative funded in initially in 1999 by the Robert Wood Johnson Foundation that is set to run through 2013. The program was developed against a backdrop of national statistics that included the following:

- From 1986 to 1996, the incarceration rate for youth ages ten to eighteen due to drug involvement increased 291 percent.

- From 1992 to 2001, juvenile arrests for drug violations increased 121 percent, while adult arrests for similar crimes grew by only 33 percent.

- Arrested adolescents are three times more likely to have used alcohol in the past month than teens overall, five

and a half times more likely to have used marijuana,
and eighteen times more likely to have used cocaine.

Treatment outcomes for adolescents in the justice system
who use drugs and alcohol indicate an overall reduction in drug-
related crime one year after they are admitted to treatment. Yet,
according to one 2007 study, estimates suggest that only 7.6
percent of young people who need treatment get it at a specialty
facility.[3]

Only a few foundations, such as the MacArthur Foundation,
the Annie E. Casey Foundation, and JEHT Foundation (which
stopped making grants in 2009), wanted anything to do with
the juvenile justice system, which was generally thought of as
difficult to work with and to change. The Robert Wood Johnson
Foundation was also leery initially. "It was a very unusual subject
for the Foundation to get involved with," acknowledges Katherine
Kraft, then a senior program officer at the Foundation and the
original architect of Reclaiming Futures. "Our movement into
juvenile justice was through the back door. If you want to deal
with adolescent treatment, you have to deal with the justice
system. That's where the kids are."

But as Robert Wood Johnson Foundation program officers
quickly discovered, the juvenile justice system is Byzantine in its
political complexity and structure. It is, for the most part, a closed
system, designed to guard the confidentiality of children and
adolescents young enough to change their lives around and not
be forever branded by their early mistakes. That confidentiality
sometimes works against the very people it is designed to protect.
Dealing with a system so closed to public scrutiny is a huge
challenge, exacerbated by the fact that it is not a single system;
rather, it is a jumble of thousands of systems, each as distinct and
unrelated as the jurisdictions under which they all serve. "Yet it is
also a system that is mandated to be in continual dialogue with the
public it serves," notes Kristin Schubert, the program officer at
the Robert Wood Johnson Foundation charged with overseeing
Reclaiming Futures. "While frustrating at times, this makes

it possible to find openings for change that, while sometimes circuitous, lead to some movement."

Adding to the challenge is the language barrier: the language of treatment isn't the language of criminal justice. The terms simply don't equate. Among the most loaded is the word "assessment." When people in the juvenile justice world talk about "assessment," they're referring to an individual's risk to society and the likelihood that he or she will commit another crime. Treatment providers use the same word to describe a client's dependency problem and risk of relapse. Reclaiming Futures had to acknowledge the validity of the two (albeit sometimes competing) definitions of "assessment" and come up with one that met its needs. Reclaiming Futures took the word to convey a whole new meaning: the assessment of an adolescent's individual strengths—be it her swim talent, love of fashion, or social skills. The program wanted to encourage strength-based treatment, which relies on adolescents' skills, to teach them ways of overcoming adversity.

"There was no end to the words we had to reconcile," says Laura Burney Nissen, the national program director, whose office at Portland State University in Oregon spent more than a year drawing up a vernacular all could agree on. "It was more around changing the culture around the terms and not just the meaning." National and local staff even hammered out an agreement about the meaning of the term "adolescent substance abuse," since, as Jeffrey Butts, a former research fellow at Chapin Hall at the University of Chicago (he is currently the executive vice president of Public/Private Ventures) and co-evaluator of Reclaiming Futures, made clear, drug use among adolescents is so pervasive that it should not be overpathologized.

—∿— The Reclaiming Futures Program

Reclaiming Futures grew out of an effort led by SAMHSA's Center for Substance Abuse Treatment in the 1990s called Juvenile Justice Integrated Treatment Networks, which included wraparound treatment, juvenile court programs, and various community youth intervention models. But the Foundation model went further. Citing the National Institute on Drug Abuse—that for every dollar spent on treatment, $4 to $7 is saved on drug-related crime—Foundation program officers zeroed in on a young population of mostly casual drug users who could be diverted from a life of crime and serious substance abuse.

Consultations with the nation's leading experts led the Foundation staff to conclude that the best way to do it was by changing the system in order to coordinate services and provide young people with evidence-based treatment programs. Unlike many initiatives in the substance-abuse field, Reclaiming Futures was not designed to test the behavioral impact of any particular intervention or treatment technique. It was, rather, an effort to design and implement a model of organizational change and system reform that could improve the juvenile justice and community response to young people with drug and alcohol problems. "The idea was to design effective community-wide responses to substance use problems of youth involved in the juvenile justice system by strengthening organizational networks, inter-agency collaboration, community leadership, resource mobilization, data sharing, family involvement, and treatment effectiveness," the Foundation's Schubert said. "In each community, a very deliberate approach was used to work across discipline-specific and agency-specific boundaries."

Accordingly, the $30 million program focused on system change. This meant bringing all the players—judges, probation officers, treatment providers, public defenders, community leaders, family members, and young people—to the table to foster a collaboration of information, resources, and databases. No money was allocated for additional treatment services (though some funds were available to train providers in new treatment practices). The program's mantra was threefold: More Treatment, Better Treatment, Getting Beyond Treatment.

It sounded simple, yet it was anything but. By opting to approach the problem through the juvenile justice system, the

Foundation was trying to influence a world noted for resistance to change. By calling for system change, it was promulgating a whole new way of doing business. Originally designed to set aside issues of guilt and innocence to resolve the problems of troubled youth, the juvenile justice system has become more punitive over the last twenty years, more of an adjunct to the adult criminal justice system. The goal of Reclaiming Futures was to restore it to its original intent and begin by tearing down the "silos" between the juvenile justice and community-based treatment systems—stand-alone bureaucracies that work independently of and, as often as not, at odds with one another.

When the call for proposals went out in early 2001, it was met with nearly 280 letters of intent from communities around the country—an unusually high number. After two years of meetings and culling through finalists, ten pilot sites, representing a geographic cross section of urban, suburban, rural, and Native American reservation communities, were chosen: Anchorage, Alaska; Seattle, Washington; Portland, Oregon; Santa Cruz, California; Chicago, Illinois; Marquette, Michigan; Dayton, Ohio; Southeastern Kentucky; the Rosebud Indian Reservation in South Dakota; and the State of New Hampshire. Each received a one-year grant of up to $250,000 to create a program that would reflect the personality of its own community and then up to $250,000 a year for four years to implement the program.

The first few years were completely experimental. As Nissen liked to say, "We were flying the airplane while we were building it," by which she meant that the ten Reclaiming Futures sites were creating their new models from the ground up, attempting to determine which youth to screen, which to assess, and what to do with them once they were identified as needing help. Reclaiming Futures settled finally on a six-step model that would begin as soon as a young person entered the juvenile justice system:

- Screening—Young people should be screened for substance abuse issues as soon as possible after entering the juvenile justice system.

- Assessment—If indicated by the initial screening, an assessment should be done using a validated measurement tool to determine the severity of substance abuse and provide information needed to craft a service plan.
- Service coordination—The different agencies and organizations that provide services should coordinate their efforts.
- Initiation—Services should begin within fourteen days of a juvenile's assessment.
- Engagement—There should be three service contacts within thirty days of the assessment.
- Completion—The group that designs the service plan should determine how much of it needs to be accomplished before it is considered complete. As a plan is completed, young people become more involved with services in the community.[4]

Although all six steps were incorporated into every site's plan, each of the sites chose which steps to emphasize and implemented them in its own manner.

Following these steps would ensure that every arrested teen was screened for drug and alcohol problems and, if needed, assessed for the severity of the problem, provided with prompt access to a treatment plan coordinated by a service team; and connected with employers, mentors, and volunteer service projects.

"You have to screen kids, assess kids for strengths as well as challenges, get them to treatment, and make sure the treatment is evidence-based," Nissen says. "You have to make sure that community and families are involved, so that when you get them out of treatment you hook them up with different activities that sustain the gains. So from the moment kids come in, they won't hemorrhage through the system."

The challenge was to create a model that could do all that, as Nissen says, "in a hundred different ways"—one that was consistent yet flexible enough to work in such disparate communities as Anchorage, Chicago, and the Lakota reservation in Rosebud, South Dakota. "Because nothing had ever been done quite like this, we had to spend the first couple of years looking at ways for how to move this very diverse group of church leaders, parents, judges, and defense attorneys, to get them to sit around the table and figure out what's the problem and what's the solution," Nissen says.

—⁓— Reclaiming Futures in Practice: Reports on Three Sites

Each of the ten communities developed and pilot-tested its own approach, some working to settle long-standing turf battles while others were addressing administrative procedures and data-sharing arrangements. They all focused on system change to improve the coordination and effectiveness of the juvenile justice and substance abuse treatment systems. And they attained varying degrees of success, as the three case studies below illustrate.

Anchorage, Alaska

Anchorage is a city of 279,000 that, despite an abundance of stylish and expensive restaurants, retains the feel of a frontier town. In the last decade, the immigrant population has grown rapidly, and the Anchorage school system now has students speaking 94 languages, from Somali to Hmong and Macedonian. Surrounded by snow-capped, rugged mountains, the city has architecture that is flat and uninspired; the Great Alaska Earthquake of 1964 demolished almost everything that came before it. Its residents describe it as a "big small town" where friends and acquaintances routinely run into one another. That's especially true in the field of criminal justice, where there's plenty to discuss. Alaska has one of the highest rates of drug and alcohol abuse in the country; in 2004–2005, it had the highest percentage of people twelve and older needing but not receiving treatment for drug abuse.[5]

So when William Hitchcock, the presiding judicial officer of Anchorage Children's Court, came across a description of the Reclaiming Futures project in 2001, he immediately recognized its potential. After twenty of years of working inside the system, he didn't have to be persuaded about the need for an integrated approach. He was deeply frustrated by what he regarded as "the endless spinning of kids through probation." He saw himself as the city's linchpin, motivated by a conviction that judges need to lead "from in front of the bench and not just behind it."

Another instrumental figure was Linda Moffitt, intake supervisor of Alaska's Department of Health and Social Services in the Division of Juvenile Justice, who has spent her entire career in Juvenile Probation, moving up from a temporary social worker in 1986 to her current position. A no-nonsense outdoorswoman who has spent time backpacking and boating above the Arctic Circle, Moffitt says she, too, was frustrated by the nonstop spinning. "What interested me was the idea of system change," she says. "You throw money at a problem for a few years, the money goes away, and then everything goes back to normal. Thankfully, that's not going to happen here."

Anchorage thought it knew all about collaboration and was perfectly positioned for the demands of Reclaiming Futures. For years, members of the Anchorage Juvenile Justice Working Group had been meeting regularly to brainstorm about how to address the problems of city youth. "We thought we worked well together, but we just sat well around the table together," Hitchcock now says, looking back. As the initiative moved into its third year, the collegiality began to fall apart, and the entire project fell into jeopardy.

The conflict came to a head over a new seven-question screening tool that asked questions such as:

- Have you ever ridden in a car driven by someone (including yourself) who was "high" or had been using alcohol or drugs?

- Do you ever use alcohol or drugs when you are by yourself, alone?

- Have you ever gotten into trouble while you were using alcohol or drugs?

If a young person answered yes to at least two of the questions, he or she was automatically referred for a more detailed assessment.

Until Reclaiming Futures came along, the thirty-five state probation officers based in Anchorage had wielded individual discretion over how referred juveniles got screened during intake. Now, suddenly, they had lost their autonomy and had been saddled with more work, as the seven-question test became a universal mandate. Its adoption would become a test in itself and take three years of struggle before being accepted—a credit, by most accounts, to Moffitt's tenacity. "For a few years, I felt like I was banging my head against the wall," she says.

Other problems emerged, including internal turf battles. A couple of different directors came and went, and a communications breakdown almost blew the entire mission off course. Treatment services for young people were being delayed, and the resistance from probation officers was thwarting program goals.

Finally, in 2005, the city's third and final project director was appointed: Tom Begich, a folksinger with a long braid down his back and a venerable Alaskan lineage (his father was Nick Begich, the Democratic congressman who disappeared in a plane over Alaska with House Majority Leader Hale Boggs in 1972; his brother is Mark Begich, the former mayor of Anchorage, who was elected to the US Senate in 2008). Begich is a dynamic figure with a lot of juvenile justice credentials. In 1997, he was national chairman of the Coalition for Juvenile Justice; from 2001 to 2005, he chaired the Alaska Juvenile Justice Advisory Committee; from 1997 to 2000, he served as community justice coordinator for the State of Alaska.

"One of the biggest difficulties we had was getting our head around the concept," Begich says, referring to the problems of enacting the Reclaiming Futures model. "We didn't know how to share resources and collaborate really well. We thought we knew. But we'd never taken the big risk of sharing money, people, and resources."

In fact, the Anchorage site was well into its third year before any young people—any clients—began being accepted. That, says Begich, is when the program started to gel. It instituted a strength-based treatment program that used positive language in its screening and assessment of adolescents, one that addressed their assets and goals and didn't simply repeat the well-worn threat, "If you keep acting like this you're never going to make it!" The way Anchorage interpreted it, strength-based treatment also meant a reliance on incentives, like movie passes, $5 gift cards, and fast food coupons, to reward positive behavior and encourage active engagement in treatment. Providers say that there's "a magic moment" that comes in treatment: if they can get a young person to a treatment center three times, they've "hooked" them.

To coordinate services, Anchorage designed a Web-based data system of real-time case management, which when it is completed will allow the city to aggregate statistics and track recidivism. It hired a mental health assessment clinician and, for the first time, began providing integrated treatment assistance for young people with multiple mental health disorders. By the time the five-year grant ended, the city was so pleased that it independently funded and commissioned an evaluation of Reclaiming Futures in Alaska. Conducted by André Rosay at the University of Alaska, Anchorage, the evaluation found that since the implementation of Reclaiming Futures, teenagers in the Anchorage juvenile system were five times more likely to complete treatment than were similarly placed teenagers before Reclaiming Futures began. The evaluation also found that members of the treatment team were collaborating to provide a consistent response and relying on better communication between all interested parties—including the youth, his or her parents, probation officer, case manager, treatment counselor, defense attorney, school staff, and "natural helper."[6]

A natural helper is an older mentor or friend who preferably arises naturally out of a young person's own life. It's a role on which Reclaiming Futures places a lot of import. Most of the sites, including Anchorage, have struggled to adopt it. But a few months ago, case manager Jerry Shough found himself sitting across the table from a new client, a heavily made up fifteen-year-old who lived with an elderly grandmother. When Shough asked if she had "a natural helper," she said no. "But of course that means nothing, the lingo changes almost daily," says Shough, a large and easy-going Alaskan whose office walls are plastered with newspaper headlines and photographs of the now former Governor Sarah Palin. "I was looking at her and her hairdo, it was an extravagant hairdo with four different shades of color. And I asked, who does your hair? It turned out she had a very strong relationship with her hairdresser. She had a standing appointment every week. She said, 'Me and my hairdresser are really good friends. We talk, we go to lunch, she's like a big sister or auntie to me.' Bingo!" The next day, Shough drove over to the salon, sat down for a haircut, and then took the stylist out for coffee. From that point on, the stylist became an integral member of the girl's treatment team.

While those kinds of stories can be told in almost every one of the ten sites, project officers in Anchorage also credit Reclaiming Futures with bringing about system change—coordinated services and widespread reform. They say that if the money from Reclaiming Futures had gone simply to treatment services, nothing lasting would have come of it. Indeed, it is system change that paved the way for several new funding sources. These include two-year $115,000 grants from the Alaska Mental Health Trust Authority, a $205,000 three-year grant from the Rasmuson Foundation, and a $120,000 three-year grant from the Alaska Division of Juvenile Justice.

"If you do it right," says Begich, "Reclaiming Futures changes everything in your community, not just juvenile justice." To nail home the point, Begich quit his fulltime post in early 2008 and assumed a voluntary position with the program. "After a certain time, we decided there wasn't need for a paid director," he says. "One of the things about proving you have system change is you don't need an executive director." The model has also proved to have legs. Steve McComb, director of State of Alaska Division of Juvenile Justice, was so impressed with the outcomes of Reclaiming Futures in Anchorage that he is preparing to take the model statewide. Universal screening of new clients is already the norm.

As for Courtney, she "graduated" from the program in September 2008, after three months of drug testing, counseling, and therapy sessions. The results, for her, are a mixed bag. She and her mother agree that she's doing "fine." At eighteen, she's working full time as a lifeguard, finishing up high school, and living with her parents. She bought a truck that's the pride of her life and has a boyfriend—the same guy, it happens, that she once stabbed. To complicate things, however, she freely offers that she resumed her daily marijuana habit as soon as she completed the program. "I knew as soon as I got out of the intensive program that I would smoke weed," she says, shrugging.

In individual terms, success, clearly, is a mixed bag. Courtney refused to attend Alcoholics Anonymous or any other twelve-step program because, as she explains, "I'm too young to go to AA. They're just old men there." Nevertheless, she maintains that she's a changed person. She no longer gravitates toward raves and other large crowds, and she has recently discovered a love of food that's helped put thirty pounds on her previously emaciated 5' 6" frame. Whatever happens, she insists she'll never go back to being the girl she used to be. "Even if I do decide to do drugs, I would never let myself go there again."

That may not sound very promising. It's not the kind of story that makes her a poster child for the kind of success envisioned by government and philanthropic fundraisers who are looking to stamp out drug abuse once and for all. It is, however, the kind of story that hints at how complex the problem is, because like most kids coming through the doors of Reclaiming Futures and other treatment programs around the country, Courtney remains at high risk. She is someone who struggles with the disease of addiction; her relapse, far from being an indication that the program has failed, is in fact a signal that more treatment is needed.

Chicago, Illinois

Lack of funding for addiction treatment became a major sticking point in Chicago, Cook County, birthplace of the world's juvenile justice system and one of the largest and most politically complex juvenile justice systems in the country. Its annual budget is enormous (in 2008, for example, the appropriation for juvenile probation and court services in Cook County was $32 million), and beside it the $250,000 a year from Reclaiming Futures appeared a mere pittance. "Frankly, it was such a small amount, it did not buy any services," says Rick Velasquez, executive director of Youth Outreach Services, the treatment provider for Reclaiming Futures Cook County.

Local resources were so strained that a third of the identified youth went missing between screening and assessment. Only one counselor was available at each of the two designated facilities, and each of them was responsible for screening and assessment. Their caseloads were overwhelming: 300 screenings a year on average, with about half of them referred for further assessment. Assessments routinely got delayed thirty days or more after screening, and the caseworker needed to leave the office for outreach, visiting young people at home to try and nudge them back in for treatment. But by then, many of the kids had disappeared and were never found—until their next arrest.

"They couldn't do anything about it because the funding provided for exactly one person at each facility to do the screenings and assessments," says James Swartz, associate professor at the Jane Addams College of Social Work at the University of Illinois at Chicago and the site's evaluator. "There was nothing more that a person could do."

The Cook County initiative focused on North Lawndale, an economically hard-pressed black neighborhood that for years has served as a real-life laboratory for academic social workers. The money from Reclaiming Futures helped to fund training for evidence-based models, as well as to provide training for staff in new interviewing techniques. But when the local site tried to create a youth advisory council, it proved difficult. "It was a very hard community to connect with, simply because there was distrust of the system," suggests Donald Robinson, director of program development for Chicago Youth Centers. "The organizations and nonprofits that serve the community, they're leery of outside groups coming in. It's been a testing ground for a lot of different initiatives that have failed. They're not going to let you just come in and do whatever you want."

Robinson, who served almost three years as Cook County's project director for Reclaiming Futures, and other leaders strove to make a partner of the nonprofit Westside Association for Community Action, one of the key players in the neighborhood. That organization, however, was stretched financially, and never had the resources or staff capacity to give Reclaiming Futures much support. Nor did it help that Reclaiming Futures was strictly about system change. "These nonprofits are struggling, they need resources," Robinson says. "And we weren't offering them any. They didn't see us as being of any help."

Adding to the difficulty, universal screening got shot down by Cook County public defenders on the ground that any negative information might wind up in the hands of the state's attorney and possibly incriminate an adolescent pre-trial. Therefore, a decision was made early on to screen young people only following adjudication and after they were diverted out of the criminal justice system.

Perhaps most troubling, the idealism of Reclaiming Futures rubbed up against a widespread cynicism and "innovation fatigue" that permeated the juvenile justice system—and not only in Cook County. "There are multiple initiatives going on," notes Velasquez, "and it wasn't like here's a new way of thinking."

In addition, Cook County did not want Reclaiming Futures to tell them what to do. "We didn't want them to come in and be prescriptive to us and say this is the way it should be," Velasquez says. "Wait a minute, *we* know how it should be. There were times they tried to do that and we pushed back." Velazquez continues, "I remember that there was something about how we should look at mentoring and community involvement. Like there was another jurisdiction with this great mentoring program and they wanted us to put that program into Cook County. Well, that wasn't going to happen. We had another set of partners, another way of doing things. Thank you but no thank you!"

According to Swartz's evaluation, Reclaiming Futures had a profound impact on the organization of probation services in Cook County. It inspired the introduction of new, quarterly meetings between the court, substance abuse, and mental health providers to discuss service coordination and to address existing service gaps. The most solid and valuable part of the program was its screening. Young people who previously would never have been recognized as having problems were suddenly being identified. "But once the kids got out of the screening process, any kind of crack they could fall through, they fell through," Swartz notes. "I looked at the data every way possible, and I could not find any indication that the program actually had an effect on kids being rearrested."

His conclusion? The young people of Chicago were, indeed, being thoroughly screened—and then released back into a world without resources. "The bottom line is that this did not achieve what the Robert Wood Johnson Foundation was hoping it would achieve," he says. "They spent a lot of time and money worrying about the front end, while the back end did not have the same attention or resources. You're fighting upstream against a system. The kids are going back into impoverished families—if they even have a family. And if they get any outpatient services at all, it's no more than one to three hours a week. So when you measure overall, this doesn't have an effect."

Santa Cruz, California

In 1999, the Santa Cruz County's Alcohol and Drug Program and its Mental Health Services were consolidated to form a single division in the Santa Cruz County Health Services Agency. The merger happened for many reasons, not least of which was to respond to a newly emerging population: the 70 percent of adolescent substance abusers with a co-existing mental health disorder, such as attention deficit disorder, bipolar disorder, or post-traumatic stress disorder. In a Catch-22 scenario, mentally ill youths and adults are sometimes turned away from drug and alcohol treatment centers, told that they have to get their depression under control before they can be treated for their addictions.

Despite the merger, true collaboration has, by most accounts, remained difficult. The two programs maintain separate databases, and there are so many inconsistencies between them that it is often extremely difficult to track the same youth through the two systems. William Manov, the treatment fellow for Reclaiming Futures in Santa Cruz* and the director of Santa Cruz County's Alcohol and Drug Program, says, "All the data is there but you have things like a list of names from Probation, say 100 kids,

---

* To keep people in the sites abreast of what was happening in the other sites, Reclaiming Futures developed a system of "fellows" based on shared interests among the sites. For example, the judges in all ten sites were considered "judicial fellows," and the treatment officials had their own fellowship. Each fellowship published a monograph on Reclaiming Futures from its perspective and a "how to" manual for others in their peer group around the country.

and now we're trying to find these kids in the Mental Health database. There are five Joe Hernandezes. Okay, now we have a date of birth, but the birthday is three days off. So matching the databases was difficult. Defining terms across the systems was difficult. Let's say we want to do an analysis of all the kids referred by Probation for treatment: How many get into treatment? How many complete treatment? There are half a dozen codes, with 'partial program completed,' 'left program,' 'transferred to another program.' These kids never follow a straight line. So which of these discharge codes do we want to count as 'completion'?"

In Santa Cruz, Reclaiming Futures was run by the county's probation department, an office that is nationally known as much for its forward-thinking philosophy—that addicted adolescents should not be locked up in Juvenile Hall—as for its embrace of yoga and acupuncture in getting kids through detox. The department is also highly aggressive and successful in its pursuit of national grants—sometimes too much so, according to evaluators, and even team members.

To satisfy all the different grant requirements, probation staff collects data on demographics, recidivism, caseloads, program outcomes, services offered, and the length of time it takes for drug and alcohol treatment to kick in after an identified adolescent enters the system. The reporting demands of so many grants can leave the department overextended, and their overlap makes it difficult to distinguish between the outcomes of an Annie E. Casey Foundation grant and a Robert Wood Johnson Foundation grant.

For Reclaiming Futures, Santa Cruz decided to focus on the 100 or so most deeply troubled adolescents coming into the system. In 2003, it introduced a harm reduction program designed specifically for youth. Known as the Seven Challenges, it reflects a break with traditional Twelve Step programs like Alcoholics Anonymous, with their starting point of total abstinence and call to a higher authority—a major obstacle for teens who, in the words of one Santa Cruz probation officer, "think *they* are the higher authority."

Few teenagers arrested under the influence of drugs or alcohol are easily persuaded that they have a substance abuse problem. Their only problem, they believe, is that they were caught. So, instead of asking kids to confront the bad things about drinking and doing drugs, the Seven Challenges takes a nonjudgmental approach and meets them "where they're at." It asks teens what they like and don't like about drugs, gets them talking about where they drink, with whom they drink, and when they do it. And what is often found is that most young people have never thought about these kinds of questions or taken the time to examine their behavior.

"Most traditional programs ask kids to only look at the cons," Manov says. "But the cons don't represent the full reality or experience of drinking or drug use for kids. This program doesn't judge you, it just says, 'Let's look at where you're at.' It respects their freedom of choice and helps them think through *whether* and *how* they want to move to the next stage." In doing so, the program measures success not only by sobriety but also by a change in the path to recovery, sometimes the mere contemplation of recovery. It is intended to sidestep the resistance and denial commonly encountered by traditional abstinence programs. Santa Cruz counselors say that, at its best, the Seven Challenges confers a degree of self-knowledge, along the lines, as Manov puts it, that "I haven't really thought about it, but my grades *have* dropped since I started using drugs, and maybe it isn't because my teachers are all jerks."

It took years for Santa Cruz County clinicians to be trained in this new model. Accustomed to working with an abstinence approach, some questioned this new way of thinking and balked at taking on additional work, especially since no funds were available for staff training, according to Yolanda Perez-Logan, assistant division director of the Santa Cruz County Probation Department and the project director of Reclaiming Futures in

Santa Cruz. But once they began observing results—admittedly, all anecdotal—they changed their mind. "What won people over was how well the kids were responding to it," explains Manov. "The kids were engaged. They were participating. They were speaking what appeared to be honestly. So many times, kids will clam up or say what they think you want to hear. The Seven Challenges really encourages some open honest examination. It may not be where you wish they were at, but that's the whole thing about it: you're starting where they are." The Seven Challenges is now the accepted model in this beachfront community.

Reclaiming Futures in Santa Cruz was plagued with a number of serious setbacks, beginning with the closure of two residential treatment programs in 2005. A year later, funding ran out for the juvenile drug court, an integral part of the local model.

The county also wasted precious time trying to implement the Global Appraisal of Individual Needs, better known as the GAIN, an assessment tool that is used by SAMSHA and strongly endorsed by the national program office. "No one here wanted to use it," says Jaime Molina, the Reclaiming Futures community fellow in Santa Cruz. "It was not a good fit for our site. For a couple years, people did it because they had to, but they didn't see the value in it. We got rid of the GAIN in 2007." (The Chicago and Anchorage sites also rejected the GAIN as being too complicated and, at three hours per child, too time-consuming.)

Santa Cruz replaced the GAIN with an assessment tool of its own design: a twenty-minute questionnaire called the Drug Grid. But if treatment providers thought this was going to solve their problems they were once again mistaken. Throughout 2007, Children's Mental Health—the department entrusted with giving the Drug Grid—used it for only 50 out of 400 incoming adolescents, reportedly because it was awaiting a validation study before testing it out on its young clients.

Despite such problems, Santa Cruz leaders say they are pleased with several outcomes of Reclaiming Futures, including a family-strengthening program imported from Los Angeles—the program links young people to recreational and cultural activities—to fulfill the pro-social component, an aspect of the Reclaiming Futures model that's dogged other sites. Cara y Corazon, translated as Face and Heart, has become popular within the Santa Cruz Latino community, attracting more than four hundred families in a two-year period.

The site is also pleased with how it ultimately measured up in its local evaluation, performed by Abram Rosenblatt, a researcher specializing in children's mental health in the Department of Psychiatry at University of California, San Francisco. In a comparison of adolescents before and after Reclaiming Futures, Rosenblatt found that young people who went through Reclaiming Futures had more contacts with Mental Health and fewer contacts with the court system.[7] "Which is exactly what you want to see," Manov says.

—∿— Reclaiming Futures in Retrospect

Jeffrey Butts, the former research fellow at Chapin Hall, and John Roman, a senior research associate at the Urban Institute, evaluated Reforming Futures. The evaluation was based on surveys, conducted in each of the sites every six months, that tracked the quality of juvenile justice and substance abuse treatment systems as reported by twenty to forty expert informants in each community.

Their evaluation, published in 2007, found that "important and significant changes" had occurred in all ten communities. These included significant improvement in twelve of the thirteen key indicators tracked in the survey, including:

- Effectiveness of treatment
- Family involvement
- The use of screening and assessment tools
- The application of client information in planning interventions for youth

Butts and Roman concluded that "Reclaiming Futures is a potentially effective method for improving a community's response to delinquency and substance abuse."[8] According to the evaluation, focus on systemic change did in fact prove a useful way of creating effective partnerships between the various players—justice agencies, treatment providers, and community groups. "We asked people, when you break it all down what really got accomplished?" Butts says. "And what they tell you is, 'The main thing is we know each other now. I know the judge. I can go talk to him.' That happened because of all that repeated face time away from the office." They noted that more research would be needed before the link between system reform and improved outcomes in individuals could be made.

The variety of approaches adopted by the sites, however, has led some to level a criticism that there was no genuine core to Reclaiming Futures. That is, since the methods for reaching the program's goals varied so widely—from improved screening to use of drug courts—was there a basic model that could be applied universally, or at least followed by other communities?

Roman, the program's co-evaluator, agrees that the initiative was unstructured, especially in its early days when the vision was admittedly general. But he regards that as positive. Such open-ended guidance can be inspirational, he notes, empowering jurisdictions to define their own agendas and make a difference as they see fit. "To have more freedom and inspiration can be the best thing," he says.

Looking at the program as a whole, Amy Singer, senior vice president of New York's Phoenix House, one of the nation's largest nonprofit substance abuse treatment programs, concludes, "It brought people together who might not otherwise have come to the table and collaborated." As one of the early proponents of Reclaiming Futures, she considers it one of her secret great accomplishments. "I've worked in treatment, and in government at probation and corrections agencies, and in a district attorney's office, and I know how limited and siloed these agencies are," she says. "The structure of Reclaiming Futures required regular meetings across different sectors. There was an emphasis in the early meetings on establishing strength-based assessments, and that's gotten into the DNA of many agencies in a way that wasn't seen before."

But did Reclaiming Futures lead to system change? It depends on what office window you're looking out of. In early 2008, Stephen Siegel, who was the Reclaiming Futures' judicial fellow and a commissioner of the California Superior Court in Santa Cruz County, was rotated out of his juvenile delinquency assignment and replaced by a number of visiting and substitute judges. His departure was followed by a steady increase in Juvenile Hall's daily population. If there had been true system change, Siegel says, the philosophy of an individual judge would make only a small difference to the system.

Others in Santa Cruz came away with a more favorable perspective, heightened after they saw the site's flow chart in the national evaluation report. It showed a spider web of departmental interactions, marked with connections and collaborations from around the county. Tangible proof came in 2008 when county funding cut off the counseling of young drug users in area schools. Three different departments put their heads together at a meeting and agreed to share money, resources, and staff in order to continue the program. "And that's when we all suddenly got it," project director Perez-Logan says. "We weren't just wasting our time meeting. That was amazing. That was system change."

"The next step," the Foundation's Schubert says, "is to take what has been learned and make it more accessible to more communities—to teach new sites how to take the Reclaiming Futures model and adapt it to their own communities." Through a partnership between government and philanthropy, Reclaiming Futures is expanding its reach. Beginning in 2007, Reclaiming Futures received funding for sixteen additional sites from the federal government's Office of Juvenile Justice and Delinquency Prevention and Center for Substance Abuse Treatment, The

Kate B. Reynolds Charitable Trust, and the Robert Wood Johnson Foundation. The Robert Wood Johnson Foundation authorized $4.5 million effective from June 2007 through December 2011 to enable the national program office to provide technical support to the new sites.

From the beginning, the concept behind Reclaiming Futures was that if you could create opportunities for open dialogue and better collaboration between agencies, you would improve outcomes for adolescent clients. The idea is not so different from the model for family therapy: better relations between parents ultimately trickle down and result in improved child behavior. "They showed they can do system change—which, by the way, is not easy," notes David Rosenbloom, the founder of Join Together, a Boston University-based organization devoted to advancing effective alcohol and drug policy, prevention, and treatment, and, since 2009, the president and CEO of the Center on Addiction and Substance Abuse at Columbia University.

This much, he says, is known: "It's very expensive to have uncoordinated activities. We waste so much money by not talking to each other. The processes they were addressing were so dysfunctional that even if all they did was to improve the communication between the agencies—if they made for a better work environment for the people within the system—I think it was worth it." "But does that prove the hypothesis that if you change the process, kids do better?" Rosenbloom asks. "I don't know whether the demonstration has gone on long enough to answer that question."

Notes

1. Office of Applied Studies, Substance Abuse and Mental Health Services Administration, Department of Health and Human Services. *Treatment Episode Data Set (TEDS) 2002: Discharges from Substance Abuse Treatment Services.* http://wwwdasis.samhsa.gov/teds02/2002_teds_rpt_d.pdf. Accessed on June 11, 2009.

2. National Institute on Alcohol Abuse and Alcoholism. *Five Year Strategic Plan for Research*, 2006. http://pubs.niaaa.nih.gov/publications /AA74/AA74.htm. Accessed on June 11, 2009.

3. Office of Applied Studies, Substance Abuse and Mental Health Services Administration, U. S. Department of Health and Human Services. *2007 National Survey on Drug Use & Health*, 2007. www.oas.samhsa .gov/nsduh/2k7nsduh/2k7Results.pdf. Accessed on June 11, 2009.

4. Pilnik, L. "Reclaiming Futures: Freeing Youth from Drugs and Crime." *Child Law Practice Online*, *27*(2), 2008.

5. Office of Applied Statistics, Substance Abuse and Mental Health Services Administration, U. S. Department of Health and Human Services. *National Survey on Drug Use and Health*, table B.21. www.oas.samhsa.gov /2k5State/AppB.htm#TabB.21. Accessed on June 11, 2009.

6. Rosay, A. B. *Selected Results from Local Evaluation of Reclaiming Futures, Anchorage, AK*. University of Anchorage Justice Center, April 2007. http://justice.uaa.alaska.edu/research/2000/0713reclaimingfutures /0713.evaluation.pdf. Accessed on June 11, 2009.

7. Rosenblatt, A. *RWJ Reclaiming Futures in Santa Cruz County: Initial Policy Report*, 2008. www.santacruzhealth.org/pdf/Reclaiming%20Futures %20SC%20Report%201.pdf. Accessed on June 12, 2009.

8. Butts, J. A., and Roman, J. *Changing Systems: Outcomes from the RWJF Reclaiming Futures Initiative on Juvenile Justice and Substance Abuse*, 2007. http://www.urban.org/publications/411551.html. Accessed on June 12, 2009.

CHAPTER 8

The College Alcohol Study

Lee Green

N oon at home on a Sunday. Stephen Guest hears a scream, a sound unlike any he has ever heard from his wife before. Responding to the urgency in her voice, he finds her in the front entryway. Two police officers wearing solemn expressions stand just beyond the open door. The male officer, repeating what he has just told Stephen's wife, does the talking. Fatal accident . . . Kristine . . . upstate New York . . . frozen lake . . . snowmobile. Yes, we're sure. No, there's no mistake. We're very sorry.

The officer speaks with conviction, but Stephen and Ellen Guest still think he has it wrong. Kristine, a junior at Quinnipiac University in southern Connecticut and at twenty the oldest of their three children, had mentioned nothing about going away for the weekend. And snowmobiling? No, that didn't sound like her.

"The first thing we did was try to call her cell phone," Stephen recalls. "When that didn't work, we started calling her friends."

The only consoling element in the rush of ensuing details was that death came so swiftly that it's unlikely Kristine suffered. Attending a big, all-night bonfire party on the lake that marks the campus boundary of Paul Smith's College in the Adirondacks, she had consented to a snowmobile ride on the ice in the predawn darkness. Joshua Rau, the twenty-year-old Paul Smith's student at the controls, seemed inebriated earlier, but now, at 4:30 in the morning, he appeared to be fine. Throttling up, he pointed the machine away from the bonfire, into the dark expanse. He was going fifty miles an hour when he plowed into a narrow spit of land that juts into the lake. The impact launched both driver and passenger. Some of the other partiers, concerned when their friends didn't return, went in search of them. They found the bodies shortly after daybreak.

Just a week earlier, the lakeside college had lost another student when Stephen Welch, driving his Toyota pickup near campus at three in the morning, veered off the road and into a culvert. Fifteen months later, two more students from the college drowned when their canoes capsized on the lake late at night.

All five deaths had one thing in common: alcohol. Welch had been drinking before he crashed his truck. The two canoeists were paddling back to campus from an island after a drinking party. Alcohol flowed at the bonfire party the night Kristine Guest died. Postmortem tests showed her blood-alcohol content was negligible, but the kid who took her out in the snowmobile was legally intoxicated.

—∿— College Drinking and the Toll It Takes

Alcohol presents risks to everyone, but the combination of alcohol and young college students enjoying newfound independence is incendiary. Many experts consider alcohol abuse to be the primary public health problem facing American college students. Some colleges seemingly have tried every imaginable approach to address the issue: mandatory alcohol education for incoming students, tougher alcohol policies, better enforcement. Perhaps the most surprising development has been an organized effort by college presidents and chancellors to reopen the question of when young people should be allowed to start drinking legally. Called the Amethyst Initiative, the movement's motivating theory holds that in the quarter century since the federal government essentially forced all states to set the age at twenty-one, college drinking has only worsened, so perhaps the age should be lowered. Since the initiative was launched in July 2008, more than 130 college and university presidents and chancellors have signed on.

The problem does indeed seem intractable. Each year, because of alcohol, the parents of some 1,700 college students in the United States experience a moment like the one Stephen and Ellen Guest endured at noon on February 6, 2005. Automobile accidents claim by far the largest share of student lives, but the culture of alcohol that characterizes most campuses can be deadly in endless varieties, each more senseless than the last. Drinkers fall from balconies, participate in drunken brawls, step in front of trains, fall face down into ponds, perish in residential fires. In March of 2008, a twenty-one-year-old Bradley University student died when a drunken lifelong friend playfully shoved him as they walked on a sidewalk, accidentally knocking him into oncoming street traffic. Every year at least a dozen students—and sometimes three times that many—simply consume so much alcohol in a night that their bodies shut down and they die from alcohol poisoning. Some suffocate on their vomit.

News of such tragedies can arrive with a knock on the door or a phone call in the middle of the night. But no matter how it comes, it is the same for every parent, a searing, unacceptable gut punch that in an instant divides their lives into Before and After. All parents say the same thing: You never get over it.

While student deaths generate headlines, lawsuits, and the birth of university task forces, alcohol extracts an array of nonfatal personal and societal tolls that range from merely annoying to traumatic—tolls that affect not just drinkers but also those around them, not just campuses but also their surroundings. From noise and litter to violence, vandalism, property damage, bodily damage, sexual aggression, and unwanted pregnancies, drinking often prompts or contributes to the most unwelcome aspects of college culture. At the most fundamental level, alcohol can insidiously undermine the university's primary mission, creating in residence halls, sorority houses, and fraternity houses conditions hostile to anyone actually trying to study.

—⚬— Henry Wechsler's "Retirement"

All of this interested Henry Wechsler. Despite numerous media appearances and great attention to his work over the past decade and a half, Wechsler isn't well known to the public. Among professionals in the field of alcohol abuse, however, the name Wechsler (pronounced Wexler) is as familiar as the name Budweiser. It is not enough to say that he was the progenitor and principal investigator of the most ambitious examination of alcohol use among American college students ever undertaken. As a highly visible advocate and defender of the College Alcohol Study, Henry Wechsler gave the project a human face, making sure his research transcended professional conferences and journals and found a wide public audience.

Perhaps because he comes off as unassuming, often displaying avuncular charm, many in the alcohol field refer to him not as Dr. Wechsler or even Wechsler but simply as Henry. The press usually refers to him as a Harvard professor, but that is inaccurate. He taught for four decades at Harvard's School of Public Health, until he retired in 2006, but he was never a professor. He was a lecturer, primarily conducting research and teaching part time. From his early thirties until he was fifty-six (1965–1988), he earned the bulk of his income not at Harvard but at the Medical Foundation, a Boston nonprofit, where he did research and became a top administrator. But it was under

Harvard's auspices that he conducted his seminal study of college drinking and made his mark.

That didn't happen until he was in his sixties, and might not have happened at all but for a serendipitous convergence of circumstances. At fifty-four, Wechsler learned that he had a form of lymphoma and stood only a fifty-fifty chance of surviving more than a few years. Treatment proved effective and his prognosis brightened, but brushing up against his mortality altered his outlook. "It made me think about what I wanted to do with the rest of my life," he says. "I decided I wanted to do only what I enjoyed doing." That meant leaving the Medical Foundation. After twenty-three years, the job had grown tiresome. What he enjoyed was studying drinking—in particular, drinking among students. Who drank? How much? How did it affect their lives? Wechsler was well grounded in the subject, having spent years examining drinking at high schools and middle schools and, later, at some thirty colleges. He embarked on that work in the late 1960s, the Age of Aquarius, with recreational drugs ascendant. "Everybody pointed to drugs as being the danger," he recalls. "I always felt that alcohol was a much more widely used substance and therefore more dangerous."

He still feels that way. "Alcohol-related deaths by far exceed drug-related deaths," he says. "Alcohol is in more widespread use, it's legal, it's traditional, and people aren't afraid of it like they are drugs that come from other countries or cultures. It's all-American, it's widely advertised, it's pushed."

But there was something else that drew him to the subject. Trained as a social psychologist (Ph.D., Harvard University, 1957), he found the study of alcohol use appealing "because it really intersects all sorts of disciplines, from genetics to psychiatric and clinical to social to political to economic, environmental. It crosses all of these lines, so it's a fascinating subject of study."

By 1992, when he was six years out from the cancer, the outlines of an ambitious project had crystallized in his mind, though he hadn't yet worked out the details. Having long since left the Medical Foundation, he found that the arc of his life had flattened. He had become a researcher in search of a project. His earlier examinations of college drinking had been geographically limited, focusing entirely on schools in New England. What was needed now to truly illuminate the full scope and nature of the problem was something much bigger, a national study that looked at a hundred or more colleges, a survey that included tens of thousands of students.

—᠆ᢍ᠆— The Birth of the College Alcohol Study

As Wechsler contemplated such matters, the Robert Wood Johnson Foundation was working through a transition of its own. Steven Schroeder had arrived in 1990 as president of the organization and wanted to tackle substance abuse, especially tobacco. "That was his real interest," says Marjorie Gutman, a senior program officer from that era. Illicit drugs would be targeted, too—you could hardly call a new portfolio Reducing Harm from Substance Abuse without including illicit drugs—but when it came to alcohol the Foundation was ambivalent. As the portfolio's priorities emerged, Gutman says, "Alcohol was not one of them."

That would change. Nancy Kaufman, a nurse specializing in public health and preventive medicine, whom Schroeder brought in as a vice president in 1991 to guide the Foundation's substance abuse efforts, reviewed the existing programming. "It was really obvious that the big thing the Foundation was missing was work in alcohol," she says—no small omission given that alcohol was "probably the number one drug of abuse for young people." As a physician, Schroeder knew the health consequences of drinking, and there was a personal hook. In college, he had lost friends in alcohol-related car accidents. Both of his sons lost friends the same way in high school. "So I had a sense that this was an important public health issue," he says.

Kaufman and Gutman knew they wanted to move forward with alcohol, and both liked the idea of focusing on college drinking. "This was an area ripe for the Foundation's involvement because the problem was escalating," Kaufman says. But how should they begin? She had been pondering that question for about a week when Gutman walked into her office holding an envelope. "Somebody has been eavesdropping on our discussions," she said. "I just got the most interesting proposal over the transom. You're not going to believe it."

Kaufman worked at the Foundation for more than a decade, but, like Gutman, she remembers that moment vividly: "She handed me Henry Wechsler's proposal to do a really scientifically sound epidemiologic study of patterns of drinking on college campuses. I almost fell over. Honestly, it was kismet."

Unbeknownst to Kaufman or Gutman, a few months earlier Wechsler had journeyed south from his home in Quincy, Massachusetts, to the Foundation's Princeton, New Jersey, offices and pitched his concept. "The next thing I knew, I had an invitation to write a grant proposal, which I did," he says. But neither Kaufman nor Gutman had attended that meeting or even knew about it. Until they received Wechsler's written submission, they hadn't even heard of him, let alone his idea.

"When we got the proposal from Henry, it was exactly what we wanted to do," Kaufman says. The staff, however, had mixed feelings, and the board of trustees was skeptical. The attitude of many, Gutman recalls, was, "'Alcohol is normal. What are we talking about here? Yeah, people have a few drinks, college kids drink. What's the big deal?'"

Further reluctance stemmed from a sense that taking on alcohol was "risky." It wasn't like taking on cocaine. Alcohol was legal. Most Americans liked it and used it. You had the weight of tradition and the entire culture against you. Moreover, to make any inroads, you had to push for policy changes, but pushing for policy changes looks a lot like lobbying, and Foundation money can't be used for that. Kaufman recalls, "The attitude was 'You already put us at risk with the tobacco stuff, now why on earth do you want to have another real risky thing going on at the same time?' That was literally said to me in the staff review meeting. But Steve [Schroeder] was all for it. He got it. He wanted to do something, and he was really the one who bolstered us up to go ahead and do this."

The 1992 grant the Robert Wood Johnson Foundation made to the Harvard University School of Public Health to enable Wechsler to conduct the College Alcohol Study totaled just under a million dollars. "Initially we just funded it as a one-off," says Gutman, who served as the project's original program officer. One grant, one survey. That was all the Foundation envisioned at the time. The idea was to generate a data set—objective, scientific evidence to define and document the problem—that could be used both inside and outside the Foundation. Inside to convince reluctant staff and board members that college drinking wasn't just a benign tradition but a menacing health problem worthy of further investment. Outside to convince universities and their surrounding communities of the same thing. "They were going to have to make some pretty significant changes" in their alcohol policies, says Kaufman, who served as Wisconsin's deputy director for public health before Schroeder recruited her to the Foundation. "I had been involved in trying to make some of those changes on the UW-Madison campus, and I knew this was not going to be a waltz."

To accomplish anything in the policy arena, says Joan Hollendonner, a former Foundation communications officer who worked extensively on the College Alcohol Study, "it's not good enough to just have a sense of the problem. You need to document and have the data to support whatever your argument is and whatever actions you might want to take."

—⚬— The Surveys

Henry Wechsler's efforts to provide that documentation would go well beyond the one-time survey originally envisioned. The results of that initial effort, published in December 1994 in the *Journal of the American Medical Association,* generated not just attention and academic debate but so much invaluable data that the project was expanded. By the time the study concluded, the Foundation had awarded Harvard not one grant but seven—four totaling $5.3 million for research surveys, three worth $1.2 million to disseminate findings. From the initial grant to the publication of the final survey data, the College Alcohol Study lasted fourteen years (1992 to 2006). It produced four distinct national surveys (in 1993, 1997, 1999, and 2001). Wechsler and his Harvard research team of epidemiologists, behavioral scientists, and biostatisticians examined the drinking patterns and practices of 50,000 students on 120 campuses in forty states. "A landmark national study," declared the *New York Times,* though not everyone was impressed. Jay Leno flippantly asked if we really needed a team of Harvard researchers to tell us that college students drink.

The Harvard surveys looked at college drinking from a variety of angles. Using lengthy questionnaires that relied on student self-reporting, the researchers explored drinking frequency and quantity, breaking down the data by, among other things, race, sex, age, religiosity, group affiliations, marital status, and living accommodations. They looked at how drinkers affect nondrinkers, how they affect the surrounding community, and how their drinking is influenced by laws and school alcohol policies. They even looked at whether the stereotype linking sports fans and drinking is accurate. (It is.) From this blizzard of information, however, the one thing that stood out—the thing that worried college officials, alarmed parents, intrigued researchers, and lit up the media—was the revelation that two in five American college students were "binge drinkers." More than two in five, actually, and the number proved unyielding. In each of the four surveys, 44 percent, give or take a few tenths, landed in the binge drinker category.

The first time Wechsler uttered this number in public, at a press conference on December 6, 1994, at the Harvard School of Public Health, the media went crazy. ABC, NBC, and CBS television networks all led their evening newscasts with the story. ABC's coverage, anchored by Peter Jennings, went on for four minutes—an eternity in commercial television news. Burness Communications, subcontracted by Harvard to coordinate and track publicity, counted 413 broadcast exposures that reached 150 million people. The wire services, newspapers throughout the nation, *Newsweek* and *Time*—everyone jumped on the story. And the coverage didn't just dominate a news cycle and then disappear. The media couldn't get enough of it, and they all wanted Wechsler. Suddenly the quiet, rumpled, office-bound academic was a rock star appearing on "20/20," "Nightline," CNN, MSNBC, and "Good Morning America. "I found myself in a state of shock as to how this became a major news item," he says.

—w— Controversy over Binge Drinking

You can't label 44 percent of America's college students binge drinkers without attracting controversy and criticism. The Harvard study generated both, and each successive wave of data brought a new wave of criticism. And each time Wechsler and his colleagues mined the data and published another article in a professional journal, which they did more than eighty times, they invited still more. Other researchers, students, college officials, individual rights advocates, and the alcohol industry all weighed in. The study used "binge" inappropriately. The study overstated the problem. Self-reporting was unreliable. The student samples at each school were too small. Wechsler was "Doctor Doom." Wechsler was "Chicken Little." Wechsler was a teetotaling neo-prohibitionist. And not just Wechsler. The Robert Wood Johnson Foundation, squarely in the crosshairs of alcohol industry sharpshooters, was labeled neo-prohibitionist, too, essentially a temperance organization.

Through it all, year after year, Wechsler stood at the center of the storm, absorbing each blow, never shrinking from the fight, giving as good as he got. It's hard to faze someone who has survived cancer, but there was more. "I had survived once before," he says. "We fled Poland on September 1, 1939, when Germany invaded. We traveled through most of Europe one step ahead of the Germans and, miraculously, came to this country." He was almost nine years old.

In any endeavor, a single choice at the beginning can alter the nature of all that follows. Wechsler made such a choice when he decided to use the term "binge drinker" to describe students who had consumed four or five drinks (four for women, five for men) "in a row" on at least one occasion within two weeks of the survey. Because the term had a much different connotation in common usage, employing it as Wechsler did guaranteed blowback. A polemic by David Hanson, a professor emeritus of sociology at the State University of New York at Potsdam with financial ties to the alcohol industry, typified the criticism. "Bingeing actually refers to a period of extended intoxication lasting at least two days during which time the drinker neglects usual life responsibilities," Hanson wrote. "That's what it means to physicians and other clinicians and that's what it tends to mean to the public as well. To refer, as Wechsler does, to consuming four drinks on an occasion (five for men) as a binge is deceptive and misleading."[1]

Wechsler wasn't the first researcher to call five drinks a binge, but doing so in the College Alcohol Study catapulted the term to common usage in academia and scientific circles. "It's widely used internationally," he says. "We did a study, finally, because we were attacked for this term, to see how it's used. Something like 80 percent of the time it's used now the way I've used it."

Not, however, at the *Journal of Studies on Alcohol,* which refused to use it. The National Institute on Alcohol Abuse and Alcoholism resisted the term and then, in early 2004, redefined it, stipulating that the drinking had to occur within a two-hour period and produce a blood alcohol concentration of 0.08 or above. William DeJong, a professor at the Boston University School of Public Health and former head of the US Department of Education's Higher Education Center for Alcohol and Other

Drug Abuse and Violence Prevention, wrote, "There is no scientific basis for focusing on this measure [binge drinking as more than five drinks for men and four for women] to the exclusion of other consumption measures; neither is there justification for labeling such consumption binge drinking, which reinforces an exaggerated view of student drinking."[2] The Inter-Association Task Force on Alcohol and Other Substance Abuse Issues, a coalition of twenty-two higher-education associations, rejected the term altogether, stating in September 2000 that binge drinking should only be "used to denote a prolonged (usually two days or more) period of intoxication." Drew Hunter, the organization's secretary, said, "Students themselves are getting tired of being portrayed negatively as a whole for the behavior of a few. What we are asking for is to define the picture accurately."

None of this daunted Wechsler. If he had to do it again, he says, he would still attach the term "binge drinking" to the five/four-drink threshold because he likes the simplicity. "The only other term for it would be 'heavy episodic drinking,'" he says, "but I think that's clumsy. It's hard to communicate with lay people that way. That's why I like 'binge drinking.' It's understandable. And I define it every time I use it."

"I think Wechsler's five/four gets to the heart of the matter," says Father Edward A. "Monk" Malloy, president of the University of Notre Dame from 1987 to 2005. "If you ask the typical student whether that's an effective standard, especially those who drink regularly, they'd say no, it's too low. But I think the standard has served very important purposes. It gives a guideline."

"Lots of administrators and students feel like that's a pretty low threshold that allows us to make more of the problem than it really is," says Toben Nelson, a social epidemiologist who worked with Wechsler at Harvard and has done extensive research on the College Alcohol Study data. "But if you set a higher threshold, you will miss the bulk of the problems" because so many students negatively affected by alcohol would fall out of the cohort.

—∿— A Father Steps In

The College Alcohol Study illuminated not just demographics but the culture of alcohol that suffuses most college campuses and the neighborhoods surrounding them. Eighteen-year-old Lynn Gordon "Gordie" Bailey got caught in an extreme manifestation of that culture, a fraternity initiation awash in alcohol and social pressure. Just four weeks into his first semester at the University of Colorado at Boulder, Bailey and twenty-six Chi Psi fraternity pledge brothers were blindfolded, taken by fraternity members to a place in the woods, presented with four bottles of whiskey and six bottles of wine, and told they couldn't leave until they drank it all. A fraternity member found Bailey passed out on the floor of the Chi Psi house the next morning. Someone called 911, but it was too late.

Bailey's stepfather, Michael Lanahan, visited the Boulder campus a few days later to face the cruel task of cleaning out his stepson's dorm room. While he was there, he met with the university's chancellor, Richard Byyny. As Lanahan tells it, "He said, 'I don't know what we're going to do about this binge drinking at college campuses.' And I said, 'With all due respect, Gordie didn't die because of binge drinking. This was because of fraternities having initiation, using alcohol, and hazing where peer pressure is involved.' And he said, 'Well, we have no control over that because the fraternities are off our real estate.' And I said, 'Well, then, I think you should resign.'"

Lanahan is a smart, no-nonsense fellow, board chairman of the company he built from the ground up, Greystone Communities, based in Irving, Texas, which develops living facilities for seniors. He's fine with talk as long as it leads to action—a solutions guy. A year after his family's tragedy, he returned to Boulder, this time as an alcohol-abuse activist talking about "leadership and how you prevent something like this." There he met with George "Hank" Brown, former United States senator and former president of the University of Northern Colorado, who had recently become president of the University of Colorado system. "What would you do if you were in my shoes?" Brown asked. For starters, Lanahan replied, he would probably convene a committee of officials and stakeholders—representatives from the governor's office, the state legislature, the local city council, police, civic associations—"and talk about things you can do to positively impact the environment here. Just to show that you're concerned about this and you're not going to let the status quo remain."

The Gordie Foundation, established by the Lanahans and Bailey's mother, Leslie, shortly after Bailey's death, focuses almost entirely on education. Informational literature, peer-to-peer educational programs, online information and resources for students and parents—it's a formidable attempt to do what seemingly all parents who lose a child to alcohol want to do: spare other families from having to endure such a tragedy or any of the other traumatic consequences of irresponsible drinking. The Lanahans speak on college campuses around the country and have produced a slick, wake-up-call feature documentary, *Haze,* chronicling their son's story and the perils of college drinking. "We're trying to be at a national level on this topic just to raise visibility," Michael says.

At the same time, Lanahan knows he's fighting a rear-guard battle. "It comes down to two issues at the end of the day, leadership and money, as so many things in our society do," he says. "Just publicity out there is not going to change this environment."

—⁓— Changing the Culture

Change this environment. That's the phrase Lanahan keeps coming back to, which puts him in concert with contemporary thinking about campus alcohol abuse. When Wechsler launched the College Alcohol Study sixteen years ago, he didn't think in those terms. But with the explosion of interest following the 1994 release of the first round of findings, he began receiving invitations from universities to speak to their administrators, faculty, health personnel, and, occasionally, students. Off he went, turning down far more requests than he accepted but visiting a number of campuses around the country. Invariably, his hosts took him to dinner, usually just off campus.

"I noticed this ring of bars and liquor stores that seemed to surround most of the campuses I went to," Wechsler recalls. That observation prompted him to expand the study. "In addition to surveying students, we sent teams of observers to every college to pick a certain number of bars and liquor stores, look at the promotions and the prices and how alcohol was being marketed."

Wechsler's whole investigatory frame had shifted. "I had been focusing on what it is about these kids—why they are drinking, how they are different from kids who aren't drinking. Seeing all those bars and liquor stores brought home the fact that the environment was as important a source of the problem as the individual. Which sometimes is forgotten. Most studies of alcohol focus on the drinker, not on the alcohol environment."

This was one of the College Alcohol Study's most important research contributions, fostering a greater recognition of the relationship between consequential drinking and the setting in which it occurs. Heavy-drinking campuses tend to be surrounded by cheap, easily available beer and liquor. "What came out of Henry's findings, at least from the Foundation's perspective, is that the way you attack the problem is by making alcohol less accessible to underage kids," says David Morse, the vice president for communications at the Robert Wood Johnson Foundation. "For example, you reduce the prevalence of drink specials around campuses—the ladies' nights, the two-for-one and three-for-one beers. You change the environment around which kids drink."

Environmental reform can take any number of other approaches, from limiting the density of alcohol outlets around campuses to stepping up enforcement of existing laws, toughening campus alcohol policies, and reducing the barrage of beer and liquor advertising to which college students are unrelentingly exposed. Unfortunately, none of this is simple. Students like to drink. Come down too hard on them and they move the party underground—one reason supporters of the Amethyst Initiative want to consider lowering the legal drinking age.

"Colleges have been asked to shoulder almost the entire burden of this problem themselves," Toben Nelson says. "The reality is that most alcohol consumed by college students is not provided by the colleges. The sources are out in the community. We haven't effectively made the case to stakeholders in the community that changes there need to happen as well."

The most powerful stakeholder is the alcohol industry, whose incentives all run in the wrong direction. Its interests lie in sustaining rather than restricting the easy availability of alcohol and in cultivating new customers. College students, who drink more than their non-college peers, represent a huge, lucrative market. The industry consistently denies that it targets underage drinkers, who drink roughly half of all alcohol consumed by college students, but the evidence belies that claim.

"Overall, I think they are committed, on the basis of survival, to trying to foster as many people drinking their product and developing brand loyalty as early in life as possible," says Notre Dame's Malloy. "That's why they do the advertising and the special events and other sorts of things, and they have been quite successful."

Beer commercials continue to appear on collegiate sports broadcasts because they provide so much revenue to the broadcast networks. Tell broadcasters you want to eliminate or even reduce alcohol advertising, says University of Oklahoma President David Boren, and "they just say, 'Well, we're not going to talk to you if you won't give us free rein on our advertising.'"

Boren says he would prefer to have no beer ads on Oklahoma's sports broadcasts, but only a third of the National Collegiate Athletic Association's member institutions have asked the organization to ban such ads. The NCAA bans ads for tobacco products, gambling, and alcoholic beverages—except beer, collegians' beverage of choice and the one responsible for the most alcohol-related problems.

—⁓— Changing the Environment versus Changing Social Norms

Though Wechsler's surveys faithfully reported collegiate America's binge drinking average stuck at about 44 percent, and though each campus's percentage remained fairly consistent through all four surveys, the numbers varied widely from one school to the next. Some schools registered in the high seventies, whereas Brigham Young University's average was zero, according to Wechsler. Between those extremes but leaning toward the high end was the University of Delaware, one of the schools that asked Wechsler to visit its campus and speak to administrators.

The meeting went badly, at least from Wechsler's perspective. Afterward, he called Nancy Kaufman at the Foundation. "I remember him saying, 'Oh, I just had this horrible, horrible experience,'" Kaufman recalls. "You could tell he was really upset."

Not upset, says Wechsler, "bemused." The university's president, David Roselle, had opened fire with both barrels, rejecting Wechsler's data, his methods, his conclusions, all of it. "He went on and on and on," Wechsler says. "I think this came as quite a shock," Kaufman says. "Most researchers don't usually go out and meet the people they've researched and give them the data back. He was not met with open arms at quite a few places. They didn't want to hear it, they didn't believe it."

Roselle, who stepped down in 2007 after a seventeen-year run, has a different recollection of the meeting. He didn't reject the data, he says, he merely challenged Wechsler and asked hard questions. "I was skeptical of the numbers," he admits. "But I'm skeptical of social scientists and survey research in general. I always have doubts about the validity of it."

Wechsler attracted plenty of criticism, but rarely was it presented to him so directly. Much of the criticism emphasized two points: (1) the study greatly exaggerated college drinking and (2) the environmental tactics Wechsler advocated were misguided. The environmental approach centered on regulating alcohol availability, price, and promotion. The most prominent alternative was one centered on changing social norms.

Conceived in the 1980s, social norms marketing, as it came to be called, grew out of the observation cited by academic researchers that students sometimes hold exaggerated beliefs about how much drinking occurs on their campus. Once students have been disabused of their false notions through education, the theory goes, they will drink less. As Alan Berkowitz, one of the pioneers of the social norms approach, wrote, "Our behavior is influenced by incorrect perceptions of how other members of our social groups think and act. . . . Thus, correcting misperceptions of group norms is likely to result in decreased problem behavior."[3]

The alcohol industry embraced the social norms approach, promoting it editorially and providing universities with grants and consulting. Anheuser-Busch underwrote the founding, in 2000, at Northern Illinois University, of the National Social Norms Resource Center, later renamed the National Social Norms Institute and moved to the University of Virginia with another grant from the brewing company.[4] The organization's first director, Michael Haines, frequently articulated a viewpoint on social norms marketing consistent with the industry perspective. "It's a contrast to authoritarian approaches that are top-down, social-control models that threaten students with punishment or the fear of death," he said. "The social-norms model, done correctly, is driven by the students themselves. It's positive, not coercive."[5]

While the US Department of Education's Higher Education Center for Alcohol and Other Drug Abuse and Violence Prevention notes that "there has not yet been definitive research on the effectiveness of social norms marketing campaigns,"[6] Wechsler's assessment is unequivocal. He sees the method as a "feel good" approach, a hollow palliative. "If it sounds too good to be true, it usually is," he says. "It makes the [college] administration happy because you're saying there's less drinking at the school than people think. It takes the heat off the alcohol industry by suggesting that alcohol isn't so much of a problem."

In the late 1990s, the Distilled Spirits Council of the United States funded a Web site for David Hanson, the professor emeritus of sociology at the State University of New York at Potsdam so critical of Wechsler's use of the term "binge."[7] Hanson's disdain for Wechsler's work went far beyond issues of terminology. In a piece titled, "Henry Wechsler: Does He Intentionally Mislead the Public About Alcohol Abuse?" he wrote, "Henry Wechsler has a reputation for publishing widely publicized studies that are later found to be weak, inadequate, or misleading."[8] Hanson didn't spare the Robert Wood Johnson Foundation, either: "Henry Wechsler has received many millions of dollars from the temperance-oriented Robert Wood Johnson Foundation and his writings have been consistently temperance-oriented."[9]

—∿— The A Matter of Degree Program

Despite his doubts about Henry Wechsler's statistics, Delaware's Roselle knew his campus had alcohol problems. For one thing, the tailgating scene at home football games "had really gotten ugly." When the Foundation asked his university to consider participating in A Matter of Degree, a demonstration program for ten campuses to test environmental interventions, he agreed to attend a meeting of candidate schools.

The Foundation's alcohol-prevention leaders, when they funded the College Alcohol Study in 1992, anticipated following up with programming to address the problems the study documented and measured. A Matter of Degree, launched in 1996 to determine whether community-university coalitions could shape an environment that would reduce college binge drinking, realized that ambition.[10] In the decade to follow, the Foundation created or collaborated in a number of prevention programs targeting underage drinking and drug use, but A Matter of Degree was really the College Alcohol Study's only direct descendent.

Only universities identified in the College Alcohol Study as heavy binge-drinking campuses were considered. "After the data came back, Henry, Marjorie Gutman, and I sat in a room and we went over the data," former Foundation vice president Kaufman says. "The schools with the highest risk stood out, and we cherry-picked those."

"We were brought together, and they went through Henry's study, and the Robert Wood Johnson people talked about the situation," Roselle recalls. "They were quite explicit that we were not going to be anonymous. I thought that was smart, because at the end of the day you're not going to be anonymous anyhow, so you might as well put out a press release and say who's involved in it." Fearful of being publicly branded as drinking schools, some universities opted out. Roselle opted in and became one of the program's strongest advocates. "He became a real force and a leader," Kaufman says. "He would get up on the podium at our meetings and say, 'You know, at first I didn't believe this. I didn't want to hear my own data.'"

Rather than eliminate tailgating, Roselle and his staff instituted a policy requiring everyone to be inside the stadium by kickoff. "If you were still outside, the gates closed and you were told to get off the property," Roselle says. "And if you didn't like that, you got arrested." Roselle says attendance at the games went up and alcohol incidents went down. "The year before we cracked down, we transported twenty-three kids from the stadium area to the hospital with alcohol poisoning. We did not transport any in subsequent years."

The University of Delaware also began notifying parents when a student "got in trouble over alcohol abuse. That was actually against federal law when we started doing it," Roselle says. "We were the first school in the country to do that. My attitude was a simple one: 'Who's going to sue us?' If someone did sue us, we would be the heroes of all the parents in America. So I said, 'Let's just do it. Damn the torpedoes.'"

That a university president would defy federal law didn't go unnoticed. Within two years, Senator John Warner of Virginia introduced a bill that changed the law, thus changing the institutional response to parents from "We knew, but we were not allowed to tell you" to "We knew, and we decided not to tell you." Most universities now notify parents.

Students may not like that change, but parents do. "There was only one parent in all the time we were doing it who decided the correct reaction was to shoot the messenger," Roselle says. He himself liked the policy because "parents have more tools than a university does. They have the checkbook and the car keys, so they can negotiate better behavior with their sons and daughters than an institution is able to do."

The nine other schools participating in the A Matter of Degree program achieved varying degrees of success. That, at least, is the opinion of Richard Yoast of the American Medical Association, who directed the program for the Foundation. The University of Nebraska-Lincoln had great leadership and produced outcomes "probably better than any of the others." The University of Iowa "ran into a more resistant student population, so things were much harder." Things were harder still at the University of Colorado at Boulder. In the program's second year, the administration announced a new policy of holding students responsible for their behavior not just on campus but off campus as well. "The students broke into a major riot," Yoast says. "The police were involved and the whole project sort of fell apart." At Florida State, Anheuser-Busch actively opposed just about everything the A Matter of Degree coalition tried to do.[11] The main reason Florida State University was allowed to stay in the program, Yoast says, was "because we thought that site would be a good template to see how the alcohol industry can destroy a project, which they did."

Overall, he says, "I think a lot of the policies the schools instituted really improved the quality of life for students. They may not have reduced binge drinking rates, but a lot of the secondhand effects of binge drinking were substantially reduced. That was attested to, from what I can see, by students and by the surrounding communities."

Changing culture is a slow business, but at the University of Oklahoma, which was not a participant in A Matter of Degree, the process got a jump start. Two weeks after Gordie Bailey's September 2004 death at the University of Colorado, a nineteen-year-old freshman named Blake Hammontree died at Oklahoma. It was unclear whether hazing occurred, but, like Bailey, Hammontree was found lifeless in a fraternity house the morning after a night of drinking at a chapter function, a victim of alcohol poisoning. That's where the similarities end. Michael Lanahan, the stepfather so frustrated by inaction at Colorado, would have lauded Oklahoma's response. "Within a week after Blake's death, I knew I was going to do something that might be deemed dramatic, a major change in policy," says Oklahoma President David Boren. He spent ten weeks conferring with the advisory committee he formed immediately after the tragedy, then announced that Oklahoma would essentially become a dry campus. Driest of all would be student residence facilities, including all fraternity houses, even though they were located off university property.

After four years as Oklahoma's governor and fifteen as a United States senator, Boren was accustomed to political heat. He expected heat now but didn't care; he had seen the Hammontree family's pain up close. "Would you want to join me and have to look a mother and father in the eye and tell them that their child died of alcohol poisoning?" he asked student and alumni groups that questioned his decision. "I just can't do that ever again unless I know we're doing everything we reasonably can."

Oklahoma completely overhauled its alcohol policies, and the new rules were tough: mandatory alcohol education programs for entering undergraduates twenty-two or under. No alcohol at fraternity or sorority recruitment events no matter where they were held. Automatic notification of parents for any alcohol violation on or off campus. Three violations triggered automatic suspension for at least one semester. The university also allocated $60,000 a year for a program it called SafeRide, which on Thursday, Friday, and Saturday nights provided students with free taxi service within the city of Norman, where the University is located.

But the main thing Boren wanted to go after was residences. The College Alcohol Study put him on to that, showing him that residence facilities were the scenes of the biggest share of binge drinking. "So our thought was, let's attack the venue," he says. "We'll never have perfection, but let's do what we can." To enforce the policy, the university makes spot checks on fifteen minutes' notice.

Student DUI arrests dropped 77 percent from 2005 to 2007, the first two years under the new policies. Underage students caught in possession of alcohol dropped 23 percent. Public intoxication decreased 74 percent the first year alone and 59 percent over two years.

Boren's approach at Oklahoma might not work at some campuses. Each university has its own culture; some student populations are more resistant than others to authoritative decrees from the administration. But when you look at campuses that have made progress, they often seem to have someone at the top who finds the status quo unacceptable and has the courage to change it.

—⟶— The Impact of the College Alcohol Survey

Any assessment of the impact of the College Alcohol Study fifteen years after its first findings were published depends on who is doing the assessing and what yardsticks they use. Wechsler himself is the first to admit a cardinal failure if the yardstick is the impact on collegiate binge drinking. "It hasn't really decreased," he concedes. "I must say, that's a real disappointment. The other disappointment is that many colleges have not been moved to try to change the environment." In the next breath, though, he points out that most universities now have alcohol education programs, many of them mandatory for incoming students. "It used to be the alcohol educator was a part-time junior person typically working in the basement of the health services building doing posters and various limited educational programs," he says. "Now this topic at most schools is handled out of the president's office, or certainly by the dean or the vice president for student affairs."

But Wechsler isn't an education guy, he's a policy guy, a change-the-environment guy. "It's the unregulated [alcohol] market that's the problem. In some instances, the market can be unregulated, but when it deals with kids, it has to be regulated," he says.

The market is in fact regulated, but only loosely. The one complaint you will never hear from college kids is that they have trouble obtaining alcohol.

Boston University's William DeJong, who worked with Wechsler at Harvard in the 1990s, has long been critical of his former colleague and his work. DeJong is quick to admit, however, that the College Alcohol Study "helped us define concretely what the scope of the problem was." It identified the highest risk students, he says, and ultimately identified the types of environments that promote heavy drinking.

"Henry served a very valuable role in putting the issue of college student drinking on more people's radar," DeJong says. "But he also became a polarizing figure in the field. As he continued to do these surveys over time, the message from him pretty consistently was 'We're not making any progress. Nothing's working.' People in the field found that to be, number one, inaccurate, and, number two, debilitating and demoralizing. The fact is that all through the 1990s and in the early part of this decade there have been schools that have installed a comprehensive approach that does feature environmental prevention, among other strategies, and have made great progress."

Father Malloy agrees. Notre Dame's alcohol environment, he claims, "is three thousand times better than it was in the 1970s. You can't get overwhelmed by the negativity of contrary examples. They're always going to be there."

With the Harvard study's final data set nearly a decade old now and becoming stale, the big picture is murky. In the absence of new data, not all experts share Malloy's optimism. George Hacker, longtime director of the Alcohol Policies Project at the Center for Science in the Public Interest, says the situation at colleges overall isn't much better today than it was when the College Alcohol Study provided the first comprehensive look at the problem. "We're talking about a legal drug that's highly available, that in some circles is highly desirable and does nice things for a lot of people. And it has a great amount of social support."

Nevertheless, Hacker adds, the Harvard study thoroughly altered the terrain. "I think it really raised the visibility of this issue of drinking on college campuses and how that affected the lives of so many young people. It brought the issue to public attention, which I think was a tremendous contribution."

Moreover, he says, it "moved the discussion away from a singular focus on the individual alcoholic or problem drinker" and "started to demonstrate the significance of having a campus surrounded by bars offering discount drink specials every night of the week, or one where other community and policy factors sort of helped to encourage heavy drinking rather than discourage it. The study showed that those issues were important and that they ought to be addressed both by the colleges and the communities in which they're located. That was a substantial change in how we viewed the nature of these problems. It raised a lot of eyebrows."

For his part, Wechsler believes that raised eyebrows are necessary, but "what will lead to a decrease" in college alcohol abuse and its collateral damage "will be more lawsuits or the threat of lawsuits." That will be more effective, he says, "than anything I write."

Wechsler turns seventy-seven this year. He has outlived Blake Hammontree and Gordie Bailey and Kristine Guest and thousands of other college kids his research sought to save. When Wechsler thinks back on it all, the things that give him a sense of pride are the things that caused the most controversy. "The term 'binge drinking' and the five/four measure—they're kind of like my trademark," he says. "If you mark a pigeon and later study bird migration, that's the mark you'll find on my birds."

Notes

1. Hanson, D. *Henry Wechsler: Does He Intentionally Mislead the Public about Alcohol Abuse?* http://alcoholfacts.org/Wechsler.html. Accessed on June 12, 2009.
2. DeJong, W. "Finding Common Ground for Effective Campus-Based Prevention." *Psychology of Addictive Behaviors*, 15, 2001, 292–296.
3. Berkowitz, A. D. *The Social Norms Approach: Theory, Research, and Annotated Bibliography*, August 2004. http://www.alanberkowitz.com/articles /social_norms.pdf. Accessed on June 12, 2009.
4. Graves, L. "The Power of Normal." *The University of Virginia Magazine*, winter 2008. http://archives.uvamagazine.org/site/c.esJNK1PIJrH /b.4745559/. Accessed on June 12, 2009.
5. Quoted in Hoover, E. "Binge Thinking." *Chronicle of Higher Education*, November 8, 2002. http://chronicle.com/free/v49/i11/11a03401.htm. Accessed on June 12, 2009.
6. Higher Education Center for Alcohol and Other Drug Abuse and Violence Prevention, US Department of Education, www.higheredcenter .org/services/assistance/faq. Accessed on June 12, 2009.
7. Hanson, D. "Disclaimer." *Alcohol: Problems and Solutions*. http://www2 .potsdam.edu/hansondj/Disclaimer.html. Accessed on June 12, 2009.
8. Hanson, D. *Henry Wechsler: Does He Intentionally Mislead the Public about Alcohol Abuse?*
9. Ibid.
10. Parker, S. "Reducing Youth Drinking: The 'A Matter of Degree' and 'Reducing Underage Drinking Through Coalitions' Programs." *To Improve Health and Health Care, Vol. VIII: The Robert Wood Johnson Anthology.* San Francisco: Jossey-Bass, 2005.
11. Gruley, B. "How One University Stumbled in Its Attack on Alcohol Abuse." *Wall Street Journal*, October 14, 2003.

Section Four
Other Programs to Improve Health and Health Care

CHAPTER 9

Overcoming Language Barriers to Care: Hablamos Juntos

Irene M. Wielawski

Editors' Introduction

Title VI of the Civil Rights Act of 1964 declared that "No person in the United States shall, on the ground of race, color, or national origin, be excluded from participation in, be denied benefits of, or be subjected to discrimination under any program or activity receiving federal financial assistance." With the passage of Medicare and Medicaid legislation in 1965 (as well the provision for community health centers in the anti-poverty program), Title VI's requirements for nondiscrimination in medical care became applicable to just about every hospital, health center, clinic, and physician in the United States. Yet for many years health care professionals did not see providing services to patients in their own language as a legal requirement, even though the immigrant population in the United States was rising rapidly. It was only in 2000 that President Clinton signed an executive order making it clear that Title VI applied to persons with limited English-language proficiency.[1]

Although the law might have been slow to recognize something as obvious as the importance of patients and health providers being able to communicate in a language they both understood, foundations, advocacy groups, and some policy makers grasped its significance much earlier. In 1991, the Robert Wood Johnson Foundation determined that reducing the social and cultural barriers to health care would be one of its objectives. To reach this objective, it developed several programs to decrease language barriers to medical services. The most significant of these was Hablamos Juntos (We Speak Together, in English translation). In this chapter, Irene Wielawski, a free-lance journalist and former investigative reporter for the *Los Angeles Times* and *Providence Journal-Bulletin,* looks at Hablamos Juntos, examining its conceptual bases, observing the program in action at two sites, and offering some thoughts—based in part on the evaluation of the program—on the challenges to language-access programs and possible ways of overcoming them.

As this chapter illustrates, even an apparently simple idea such as providing Spanish-English interpretation can run into practical implementation problems. Reducing social and cultural barriers to care—including language barriers—requires thoughtful, sophisticated, and multifaceted approaches. Perhaps the best illustration of the importance of understanding and working within the appropriate cultural context is found in Anne Fadiman's book *The Spirit Catches You and You Fall Down,* the real-life story of how the great cultural gap between caring, well-meaning physicians and the parents of an epileptic Hmong girl led to a tragic series of misunderstandings.[2] As Wielawski observes, the Foundation has learned from Hablamos Juntos and has adopted approaches to ensuring better communication between providers and patients in the context of its efforts to improve the quality of health care and reduce the inequalities in accessing it.

Notes

1. Jellinek, P. S., and Isaacs, S. L. *Overcoming Language Barriers to Health Care.* Public policy case study. Los Angeles: The California Endowment, July 2007.
2. Fadiman, A. *The Spirit Catches You and You Fall Down.* New York: Noonday Press, 1997.

Imagine lying in a hospital room—anxious, uncomfortable, hoping for good news, fearing the worst. Now imagine all the people you have to deal with during your hospital stay. They include the doctors and nurses who stop in to take your vital signs, feel your skin, listen to your heartbeat, probe the sore places, move your limbs, and otherwise work over your body. Add to the crowd therapists, phlebotomists, x-ray technicians, pharmacists, transport and food service workers, and perhaps an aide to help you with bathing and other personal needs. Now imagine that the hospital you've landed in is in Ecuador, Cambodia, or Tajikistan and that most of the people caring for you don't know enough English to explain what they're doing or grasp what you're trying to tell them. Are you allergic to penicillin? Taking blood thinners? Prone to anesthesia reactions? Immunosuppressed?

For the majority of English-speaking Americans, this would be a rare experience—the result of an accident or a sudden illness while abroad. But for a growing number of immigrants residing in the United States this is the norm. Our hospitals don't routinely provide interpreters at the bedside, though law and regulation say they should. And when interpreters are on hand, their level of skill can vary greatly, and their use by clinicians is often erratic, even at the most progressive medical centers.

Considering what a challenge it can be for many Americans fluent in English to find their way in a busy hospital, provide a cogent medical history, or work through an insurance issue, it's not hard to grasp the impact on patients unable to communicate adequately in English and possibly raised in a different medical culture. There are no definitive data, but advocates say people with limited English proficiency often act similarly to uninsured people who delay care and fail to follow up on medication and other recommended treatments.

The situation has consequences for health care quality and cost in the United States health care system. Studies show that language and cultural misunderstandings can lead to misdiagnosis and flawed treatment. Patients who can't understand English well enough to follow self-care instructions are more likely to suffer harmful and costly complications. Even when individual patients aren't significantly harmed, experts say, the cumulative lapses, delays, and confusion resulting from missed or misunderstood messages undermine national efforts to improve health system performance and population health.[1]

The diversity of languages and cultures threaded through the American tapestry is vast indeed. In New York City's borough of Queens, for example, it is estimated that 138 languages are spoken. In California, 43 percent of the population speaks languages other than English at home.[2] Nationally, 18 percent of the population, or 47 million people, speak a different language at home, and of this group 20 million, or about 7 percent of United States residents, cannot function in English.[3] Logically, language services that facilitate communication between health care providers and non-English-speaking patients ought to be a win-win-win for patients, providers, and the system. Practically, though, how can hospitals, clinics, doctors' offices, nursing homes, home care agencies, pharmacies, testing labs, and all the other entities that make up our health care system accomplish this?

This question attracted the attention of the Robert Wood Johnson Foundation, which responded with what it thought was a tightly focused demonstration program to make the business case for investments by health care organizations in linguistic services. Called Hablamos Juntos, Spanish for We Speak Together, the undertaking was authorized to run from 2001 to 2005 with $18.5 million in funding, and was then reauthorized for three years with an additional $5.4 million (this was reduced by $3 million to fund a new program called Speaking Together). Focused on the linguistic needs of Spanish speakers, the nation's fastest-growing minority group, Hablamos Juntos had two main goals: to show that investments in interpreters, multilingual signage, and other aids to patients with language barriers were cost effective, and that they improved health care access and quality.[4, 5]

Grantees carried out many useful activities, but the program as a whole was unable to demonstrate either cost effectiveness or improvements in health care access and quality for patients with limited English proficiency, according to the program's evaluators. Instead, the program demonstrated that effective communication has more layers than an onion and transcends words. It found communication deficits that go far beyond language incompatibility and have implications for high-quality medical practice across the full spectrum of patients. And it identified weakness in some of the assumptions driving policy and national debate in this area, highlighting the need for more research and better data. These may not have been the lessons that the Robert Wood Johnson Foundation set out to extract from its experiment, but they are nonetheless valuable for being unexpected.

—∼— Anything New Here?

Language diversity among patients is hardly a twenty-first-century phenomenon in this nation of immigrants. Health care workers can recite stories about the strategies they've used to elicit information from non-English-speaking patients. And every immigrant, even those now acculturated and fully bilingual, can recall early experiences when their inability to communicate with medical personnel was a source of anxiety and misunderstanding.

Health care professionals and institutions have coped in various ways over the years, frequently relying on family members, including children, to translate for non-English-speaking patients. Other ad-hoc translators have included community volunteers and bilingual employees of the hospital or the doctor's office. Health care organizations routinely kept lists of employees' foreign language skills so they could be called upon by clinical staff in a pinch. Some clinicians have relied upon their school Spanish or Russian or Chinese to patch together dialogues with patients. Still others, referred to by linguistic experts as "heritage speakers," have used the language of their childhood to reach patients with whom they shared ethnic backgrounds.

None of these communication methods is considered ideal. John Prescott, an emergency room physician who is now chief academic officer for the Association of American Medical Colleges, recalls working in a West Virginia hospital that lacked interpreters and having to press a traumatized five-year-old into service in order to obtain critically important information about the boy's injured parents. Prescott's memory of doing so is a painful one, although assuaged by the greater urgency of saving the child's parents. In this way, catch-as-catch-can communication with patients of limited English proficiency became engrained in American medical culture, and seemed to suffice, especially over the many years when acute illness and injury largely defined the clinical encounter. If a patient was bleeding profusely or writhing from the pain of bone fractures, conversation necessarily took a back seat to action.

As for follow up care, there simply wasn't that much to talk about. Until fairly recently, patients stayed in the hospital until they were well enough to resume their lives and livelihood. There were few effective medicines to correct the faults in metabolism or biochemistry that undermine health over time. And most patients didn't need a detailed discharge order to tell them what they already knew from their mothers and grandmothers: stay warm, eat nourishing food, and take it easy.

It's a different world today. Take, for example, the modern hospitalization experience. People today tend to be admitted only for serious illness or injury, and discharged as quickly as medically possible, shifting the recuperative burden onto patients and their families. Patients typically go home from a hospital or surgical center with many pages of instructions for self-care that can include complicated drug therapies, special diet and exercise regimens, and the use of sophisticated assistive devices—underscoring the need for effective and ongoing communication with patients as they cope with chronic illness.

The mortality picture also is very different from a century ago. Most people alive now will die from complications of one or more chronic conditions, such as cardiovascular disease. A breakdown of current national health care spending illustrates this trend. Of the $2.2 trillion in 2007 expenditures, an estimated three-quarters was spent on chronic illness. This staggering proportion has given impetus to the movement for so-called patient-centered care, in which everyone works together to help patients achieve optimum self-care, thereby, it is hoped, improving overall population health and reducing costs from exacerbations of illness. If a child hospitalized for asthma needs follow-up monitoring by the school nurse, the hospital, school, and family collaborate to make that happen. If a diabetic's blood sugars remain high, nurse educators and dieticians step in to help the patient achieve control and avoid debilitating and costly kidney, eye, and circulatory complications.

"When you look at where our health care costs are going, you have to also consider that we have an aging population with an accumulation of behaviors that have health and financial consequences," says Yolanda Partida, a health policy researcher at the University of California, San Francisco, and a management consultant in Fresno, California, who served as the national program director for Hablamos Juntos. "Almost every chronic condition—diabetes, asthma, heart disease—is about what the patient does or doesn't do behaviorally. They have to understand the connection." In this twenty-first-century context, rudimentary provider-patient dialogues based on half-forgotten language studies, child translators, or a handy bilingual colleague have come under scrutiny. The Hablamos Juntos experiment sought to raise the communication to a professional level with specially trained bedside and telephone interpreters as well as better print materials that went beyond literal translation to incorporate nuances of Latino culture.

—⚬— Legal Mandates

A body of laws, policies, and standards developed by professional organizations define the obligations of health care organizations to ensure that patients with limited English proficiency have access to health care equal to that of English-speaking patients. This regulatory history is not without controversy. The push to address linguistic barriers for immigrant patients as well as issues of cultural sensitivity in health care delivery competes for priority with many other deficits in the American health care system. Mandates have seesawed somewhat over the years, compliance has lagged, and enforcement is generally lax, observers say.

The main platform for language access regulation and policy is the Civil Rights Act of 1964, specifically Title VI, which prohibits discrimination on the basis of "race, color, or national origin." Title VI is binding on entities that receive federal funding, which includes virtually all health care organizations through their participation in Medicare and Medicaid and receipt of government grants for research and public health services.[6]

Title VI's applicability to patients with limited English proficiency has emerged through presidential decrees and agency memoranda. The Department of Health and Human Services (HHS) made the link to language explicit in 1980 with an advisory stating, "No person may be subjected to discrimination on the basis of national origin in health and human services programs because they have a primary language other than English."[7] In 2000, President Bill Clinton signed Executive Order 13166, directing federal agencies to review all programs to ensure that people with limited English proficiency had equal access. The HHS Office of Civil Rights followed up with guidelines for health care organizations, including obligations to assess language needs in their communities, develop written policies governing language access, train staff to implement these policies, and create systems of monitoring compliance. The guidelines were softened during the administration of President George W. Bush through the addition of four mitigating factors to reduce compliance obligations and costs for small health care enterprises.[8] State law also comes into play, but there's little uniformity. Alice Chen and colleagues, reporting in the *Journal of General Internal Medicine,* describe a "haphazard patchwork of legal obligations" that varies "from state to state, from language to language, from condition to condition, and from institution to institution."[9]

Complicating the landscape even further is the fact that health insurers don't reimburse for language services in most states, putting the cost of compliance—estimated in 2002 at $268 million annually[10]—on the backs of providers and, indirectly through higher fees, on patients and taxpayers. Complaints from provider organizations, such as the American Medical Association, resulted in federal authorization for reimbursement for interpreters provided to patients covered by Medicaid and the State Children's Health Insurance Program (CHIP). But states must match the money to activate this option, and only a dozen states and the District of Columbia have opted to do so. Significantly, populous states with the largest proportion of limited English speakers—California, New York, and Texas—have not.[11]

—ᨁ— Hablamos Juntos Takes Shape

Staff members at the Robert Wood Johnson Foundation had been concerned for some time about disparities in health care for certain racial and ethnic groups compared with whites. Initially, the Foundation, like other philanthropies, sought to address these disparities by targeting broader-based barriers to health care such as lack of health insurance and a paucity of local health services. Many of the Foundation's investments in the 1980s and 1990s—for example, school-based health centers, programs to expand health care services through free clinics, and outreach efforts to enroll eligible people in publicly financed health care programs—benefited ethnic and racial minority groups primarily, but the criteria for inclusion were mostly financial. The thinking in philanthropic circles was influenced by public concern over gaps in the nation's health insurance system and the inability of many people to pay for medical services. This also drove the political agenda; a campaign promise of universal health coverage helped Bill Clinton gain the White House in 1992.

But could insurance—or the lack of it—entirely account for statistics showing that babies in certain minority groups were at unusually high risk of dying in the first year of life and, if they survived, were likely to have a shorter life span than white babies? Could it explain differences in the rate of medical diagnostic tests and preventive care provided to minority versus white patients? Could it justify higher than average rates of amputations among minority patients for complications of diabetes?

In 1991, the Robert Wood Johnson Foundation made reducing social and cultural barriers to care one of its priorities, and launched several programs to address this directly. Among the most noteworthy were Projecto HEAL and Opening Doors.[12] Projecto HEAL (Health Empowerment, Access, and Leadership), or, more formally, the Program to Address Sociocultural Barriers to Health Care in Hispanic Communities, was a $3 million program funded in 1992 that enabled eight communities to address health issues that they themselves determined as priorities. That same year, the Robert Wood Johnson Foundation joined forces with The Henry J. Kaiser Family Foundation in mounting a $5.5 million program ($1.5 million from Kaiser, $4 million from Robert Wood Johnson), called Opening Doors: Reducing Sociocultural Barriers to Health Care. According to a report on the program, between 1994, when implementation began, and 1998, Opening Doors identified a perception among minority patients across all twenty-three sites that health care personnel do not respect them, as evidenced by the absence of "active listening" (nodding, smiling, note taking, and other responsive behavior when patients described symptoms or medical history), poor eye contact, and deficiencies in basic courtesy such as addressing patients as Mr. or Mrs.[13] The grantees were able to improve conditions for specific groups of ethnic and minority patients in their communities, but the program offered little direction for system-wide improvements in language access and cultural sensitivity.

Hablamos Juntos took shape in 2001 amid ferment over emerging research showing that even when insurance coverage is comparable, patients from racial and ethnic minority groups receive lower quality care than whites. The Hablamos Juntos design team at the Foundation decided to focus on language barriers and the effectiveness of remedies such as interpreters, universally understood signage, and multilingual printed materials. Discussion at the Foundation centered on the needs of Latinos, whose numbers had risen more than 50 percent between 1990 and 2000 to 35.3 million people, or 12.5 percent of the US population. This became the genesis of Hablamos Juntos' singular focus on Spanish-speaking patients as a group from which solutions could be extrapolated to other ethnic and language groups, according to Pam Dickson, assistant vice president of the Foundation's health care group.

"There was clearly a correlation between language discordance and poor quality of care," Dickson says. "At the time, we at the Foundation were operating on the theory that a good role for us to play was as a supporter of demonstration projects. We felt the ideas would be adopted by health care organizations as a result of demonstrated competency." To achieve that result, the Hablamos Juntos call for proposals stressed the importance of designing cost-effective solutions to encourage investment by providers in language services. Hablamos Juntos grantees were charged with developing and testing systems of medical interpretation, signage, and print materials in a variety of health care settings, and gathering data on cost and patients' experience in order to answer questions about affordability and Latinos' access to quality health care.[14]

Eligibility was restricted to health care organizations that served a Latino population of at least 10,000 and that had grown by at least 50 percent between 1990 and 2000. The sites selected for the experiment were Birmingham, Alabama; Los Angeles, California; Grand Island, Nebraska; Philadelphia, Pennsylvania; Providence, Rhode Island; Greenville, South Carolina; Memphis, Tennessee; Fort Worth, Texas; Falls Church, Virginia; and Olympia, Washington. Each site initially received $150,000 to fund a year's worth of planning and organizational work, including finding community partners, cataloguing existing resources, and identifying signage and print material needs.

A two-year implementation phase, with $850,000 per site, began in 2003. That's when things got complicated, in part because of the specific questions Hablamos Juntos was created to answer, but also because of questions about health care communication in general. The first year of implementation, 2003, came on the heels of the release of a report by the Institute of Medicine (IOM) titled Unequal Treatment: Confronting Racial and Ethnic Disparities in Health Care.[15] Based on a review of more than 100 studies of quality variations in health and health care for ethnic and racial minorities, the IOM report concluded that these disparities had many causes.

Some were intrinsic to the patients themselves; for example, the report cited evidence of variations in drug efficacy in some racial and ethnic populations, and a tendency to avoid seeking care or reject doctors' advice. But stronger evidence indicted wide-ranging and deeply engrained deficiencies in the American health care system, including fragmentation of services and the linguistic barriers that Hablamos Juntos grantees were trying to overcome. Human factors also contributed to disparities, the IOM found, including prejudicial attitudes among some medical personnel or uncertainty about how to evaluate symptoms in patients who couldn't speak English. This tangle of factors and the difficulty of teasing out any one of them for meaningful experimentation challenged Hablamos Juntos grantees.

Collectively, the sites tackled many language-related issues, including training and certification of medical interpreters, deploying them effectively in health care settings, and using universal symbols to improve signage. The sites, however, had almost nothing in common. Some projects took place in large hospitals, others in small community organizations with limited resources. Two grantees were Medicaid health plans that provided no direct patient care services. Some sites focused exclusively on technical aspects of language access, such as how to bring video and telephone-assisted interpretation to geographically scattered health care organizations. Others probed psychosocial, organizational, economic, and legal dimensions of linguistic access.

There was also great variability in the population served—Latinos—resulting from the many nationalities in that demographic group. "What we learned from Hablamos Juntos is we had ten different projects addressing different populations in different locations," says Debra Perez, a senior program officer in the Foundation's research and evaluation department. "There wasn't a uniform way of assessing the interpreter services from one site to another."

While individual sites made progress toward goals within their own institutions, Hablamos Juntos as a program did not prove the business case for interpreter services. Costs were significant, with insufficient evidence of improved clinical efficiency, health outcomes, and patient satisfaction to offset them, according to an evaluation completed by the RAND Corporation in March 2007. The evaluation team, led by Leo Morales of the University of California, Los Angeles, found "only a few positive effects on patients," which the evaluators attributed partly to the experiment's short duration.[16] The evaluators also faulted leadership for allowing sites to pursue agendas that were "too ambitious for the time and resources available." In successor programs, such as Speaking Together, the Foundation addressed the conceptual flaws that the evaluation revealed. But if cross-site comparisons had to be jettisoned because of site-to-site variability, this was also the experiment's most interesting aspect. The experiences of two Hablamos Juntos grantees help illustrate this diversity of perspective among grantees united primarily by their commitment to improve the health and health care of Spanish-speaking patients.

—∿— Temple University Health System
Philadelphia, Pennsylvania

There's nothing gentrified about North Philadelphia, the area that surrounds the Temple University Health System. Here, the city's distinctive orange-tinged brick row houses feature iron bars on the lower windows; parking lots are surrounded by twelve-foot-high chain link fence and razor wire; and the most ubiquitous businesses are check-cashing and pawn shops. Gritty and dangerous after dark, it is home to predominantly working-class and unemployed Philadelphians, many of them immigrants.

A generation ago, they were Polish and Irish, living alongside the African-Americans whose presence in the area predates the Civil War. Now they're mostly Puerto Rican, though there are clusters of Cubans and Dominicans, and community leaders say the Mexicans are starting to move in. Temple's hospitals— Temple University Hospital, the system's flagship academic medical center, and two affiliated community hospitals—began noticing an increase in Spanish-speaking patients in the mid-1990s. Used to a patient mix of about half white and half black, most of them English-speaking, the newcomers unsettled business as usual at the Temple hospitals. "Our doctors and nurses began complaining about communication problems and expressing a need for language services," recalls Charles Soltoff, an associate vice president for marketing and principal investigator on the Hablamos Juntos grant.

The Temple system supports teaching and research for the Temple University School of Medicine while serving as Philadelphia's primary safety net provider, continuing a mission established by its founders in 1892 to provide care regardless of patients' race, nationality, or creed. But in today's climate, with growing numbers of uninsured patients, the mission has left Temple chronically short on capital.

"We're always challenged financially and there's a lot of internal competition for resources," says Soltoff, who nevertheless began discussions with Latino community leaders about ways to improve communication between Spanish-speaking patients and Temple clinicians. The discussions led Soltoff to develop a marketing plan with the twofold purpose of improving the Temple system's interactions with Spanish-speaking patients and cementing the loyalty of Philadelphia's growing Latino market. As part of the plan, he asked Temple's administrative leaders to consider investing in interpreters. "It was clear," Soltoff says, "that the Latino population was going to be served exclusively through our emergency room if we didn't do something."

In researching how other hospitals had responded to patients with limited English proficiency, Soltoff came upon the Hablamos Juntos call for proposals. "I read it and thought, 'Wow, this is just like my plan!'" He got the go-ahead to apply for a grant from his CEO, Joseph W. "Chip" Marshall III (who retired in 2008). "Chip's okay told me we were making a permanent commitment to interpreters, because he was opposed to grants unless they could be made a part of the core mission of the hospital." Marshall recalls being impressed with the Hablamos Juntos concept but not its focus on the linguistic needs of a single minority group. He instructed staff to think bigger.

"I told them it can't just be for Spanish speakers, it has to be for all languages and communication issues," Marshall says. "The idea was to get people at Temple focused on fundamentally changing the way we deliver care and clear away the excuses for not doing so. The Hablamos Juntos grant enabled us to kick-start that process, but it was not going to end just because the grant ended."

Lucky thing, because the Hablamos Juntos part of Temple's experience turned out to be three steps forward and two back and marked by disagreement and tension over the best use of interpreters that linger to this day. The Temple team chronicled some of this in a gently humorous pamphlet called *Confessions of a Linguistically Challenged Health System.*[17]

On the positive side, the Hablamos Juntos grant helped Temple hire in-house interpreters, promote better use of existing telephone-based interpretation services, improve the quality of translation of written materials, and adapt institutional policy to promote language access. Temple also developed its own training curriculum and proficiency standards for interpreters, after deciding that available academic and commercial programs were not suitable. Credentialing as a medical interpreter at Temple today requires forty-five hours of classroom training plus ongoing in-service sessions, observation, and practice.

The training includes lectures on physiology and medical terminology as well as on cultural diversity among Latinos, who may use different words or home remedies depending upon what country they're from. These variations based on nationality can be significant in a health care setting. For example, the word *constipación* when used by Puerto Ricans, Dominicans, and Cubans means what it sounds like in English: constipation. But this is a false cognate, used widely by Latinos from the Caribbean region possibly because of their historically close interactions with English speakers. The actual Spanish word for constipation is *estreñimiento.* And when Mexicans say *constipación*, notes Raquel Diaz, Temple's manager of interpreter training, they're describing nasal congestion.

Temple's interpreters pass extensive written and oral exams to demonstrate comprehensive knowledge of these nuances of usage. All the more bitter, then, their initial Hablamos Juntos experience: almost no one called on their expertise. In all the work to prepare Temple for interpreters, including garnering support from the system's top executives and administrators as well as Latino community leaders, no one thought to bring front-line clinical staff into the discussions. "We took away some real lessons from Hablamos Juntos," says Deborah Rosen, director of health care outreach for Temple, which oversees the current interpreter program. "We thought interpreters would be embraced with open arms—like 'Where have you been all my life?' It really didn't happen that way."

Instead, the four interpreters hired under the grant and assigned to the emergency rooms and maternity units—locations where Hablamos Juntos leaders thought they would be most needed—were initially ignored by the medical staff, who continued to rely on family members or their own language skills to communicate with Spanish-speaking patients. Even when the interpreters were called upon, protocols limited their effectiveness. They were not allowed to respond on a need basis throughout the hospital, but had to remain in their assigned locations—ER or maternity—even if there was no work to do. Also, they were not allowed to break away from an ongoing interpretation to answer a new page. This differed from standard clinical protocol, where pages must be answered promptly, and irritated medical staff, who thought the interpreters should have to operate like others on the clinical staff. (One reason that Temple restricted interpreters to fixed locations was to satisfy data collection requirements under the Hablamos Juntos grant. If the interpreters had been on a hospital-wide dispatch and triage system—as they are today—collecting data on patients' health status, length of hospitalization, satisfaction, and so on would have been impossible.)

The untested assumption of Hablamos Juntos—that medical staff would welcome the interpreters—led to tensions at Temple and a difficult work environment for the four interpreters hired under the grant. "They were asked to do things that were out of the scope of practice for an interpreter, like hold the leg of a woman in labor or push a gurney," Rosen recalls. "We had to tell the providers that this was not an appropriate role for the interpreter, but it was not uncommon for them to respond disdainfully, saying things like 'Why can't they do something more useful?

Why can't they answer the phone or do callbacks to non-English speaking patients?'"

Tension resulting from these early misunderstandings about purpose and function persisted after the Hablamos Juntos grant ended in 2005. Temple revamped its interpreter program, and today use of interpreters is mandated under risk-management and quality protocols. All staff must use in-house interpreters, agency interpreters who conform to quality standards, or telephone interpretation services if patients can't speak English or simply prefer to speak in their native language. The protocols prohibit a physician or clinician who speaks the patient's language from interpreting unless he or she has passed a test for language proficiency and is credentialed as a dual-role medical interpreter, according to Rosen. The Temple system has thirty-five dual-role employees augmenting a staff of ten full-time interpreters.

Annemarie Martin-Boyan, an attorney for the hospital, puts the rationale bluntly: "People die if you can't communicate with them. From my point of view, I don't want to deal with the complaints and litigation that can come out of a failure in this." Robert Pezzoli, former executive vice president of the Temple system, makes the same point, but anchors his thinking in the medical school precept "First do no harm." Pezzoli says, "I look at our interpreter services as an investment rather than a cost, because if we can't communicate effectively with our patients and their families, it becomes a risk."

But practical questions continue to be raised, related to resources and efficiency both in Temple's hospitals and among community-based practitioners located in forty-eight offices belonging to Temple Physicians, Inc., a subsidiary of Temple Health Systems. The ninety-five physicians receive compensation tied to productivity, making the use of interpreters a potential financial liability. "Working with a translator or a telephone language line slows things considerably," says Eric Mankin, CEO of Temple Physicians. "It takes time to find an interpreter and get him or her in the room, or alternatively to get the language line on the phone."

Mankin doesn't recall any physician in the group expressing reluctance to follow translation guidelines because of personal income concerns, but adds that productivity pressures are only one complicating factor. Not all patients welcome interpreters—a finding of the Hablamos Juntos evaluation across all sites. Some refuse their services, Mankin says, preferring family members. Mindful of the policies of their parent company, as well as federal and state mandates pertaining to language access, the Temple Physicians group now asks these patients to sign a waiver, acknowledging the offer—and their refusal—of an interpreter.

Mankin worries about the cumulative effect of such awkward and legalistic procedures on subtler aspects of patient-provider communication. "Ninety percent of diagnosis comes from the patient's story, which you get by talking and asking questions, but also through nuance and body language," Mankin says. "You lose a lot of nuance with interpreters. And it's hard to convey empathy, which is very important. Really, how can you empathize through a translator?"

Overall, however, the positives of providing interpreter services outweigh the negatives, Temple clinicians say. "The interpreters are able to provide clear answers and interpret cultural differences," Ernie Bertha, director of pediatric emergency services, said in an interview for a Foundation Grant Results Report in 2007. "Our care becomes much warmer, more personal, more personable."[18]

The manager of Temple's interpreters, Angel Pagan, sees their role in health care settings as still evolving. Now, their value is measured mostly in terms of improved clinical communication and better relations with Philadelphia's Latinos and other patients with limited English proficiency. In time, Pagan believes interpreters will also prove cost-effective, as public and private insurers penalize providers for inefficiency and errors. "Right now you have to look at this as the right thing to do for patients and for medical care quality, because you can't prove a direct return on investment," Pagan says. "But I come from a managed care background and I can tell you if you have a post-surgical patient and care or testing is delayed due to communication failure, you're not going to get paid for that extra day in the hospital."

—⁓— Molina Healthcare
Long Beach, California

Molina Healthcare is exactly the kind of managed care health plan that Angel Pagan had in mind when he predicted that interpreters would eventually be seen by health care organizations as a worthwhile investment. According to Molina's calculations, its version of interpreter services saved the for-profit company more than $1 million in 2008 simply by guiding patients to timely and appropriate health care services.

Unlike the Temple health system, Molina provides little direct care. Rather, it contracts with hospitals, physicians, and other health care professionals to provide care to its members, all of whom are covered by Medicaid, CHIP, or a combination of Medicaid and Medicare. So from the outset Molina's approach to the Hablamos Juntos challenge to improve language access was different from Temple's. This was partly due to the health plan's location in Southern California and partly to the mission established by its founder, the late C. David Molina. Molina was a public hospital emergency room doctor who wanted to improve primary and preventive care for poor residents of his community, many of them Latino. Molina's children now run the health plan; his daughter, Martha Bernadett, a physician and Molina Healthcare's executive vice president for research and innovation, was principal investigator on the Hablamos Juntos grant.

"Serving the economically disadvantaged is our main niche, but we also have members who need help to overcome language or cultural barriers," says Bernadett, noting that 60 percent of the membership is Latino. "Initially, we were planning to train interpreters and translate patient education literature. But we were saved from that by the grant's very valuable requirement that we first do a needs assessment."

The assessment revealed surprisingly negative feedback about interpreters. Bernadett says the Latinos surveyed overwhelmingly did not trust lay people to represent them or get their doctor's message right. "The responses we got were comments like 'Interpreters make mistakes. That's why I like to bring my cousin or my aunt or my brother-in-law.' And they told us about actual experiences with mistakes that interpreters had made," Bernadett recalls. "When you questioned them closer about it, you'd discover it wasn't really a big mistake, but the patient thought it was."

Molina's Hablamos Juntos team analyzed the responses in the context of Latino cultural values, which accord high esteem to doctors and nurses. It led them to abandon the translation idea and substitute a twenty-four-hour advice telephone line staffed by bilingual nurses. Called TeleSalud/Nurse Advice, the service was launched in 2004. Unlike Temple's interpreters, who serve as communication intermediaries between patients and providers, TeleSalud's Spanish-speaking nurses operate as clinicians, advising callers on self-care for minor illnesses and injuries, while directing callers with more serious symptoms to their physician's offices or the nearest emergency room.

In launching TeleSalud, Molina drew lessons from a previous, unsatisfactory experience with a commercial nurse hotline. This outsourced advice line initially seemed to be an instant success with Molina Healthcare members; data from the vendor showed a steady increase in use, according to Bernadett. But a closer look at the data revealed a startling anomaly. Only 2 percent of callers to the toll-free advice line were being connected to Spanish-speaking nurses. This made no sense in light of Molina's overwhelmingly Latino membership. "There was clearly an access issue going on," Bernadett says. "After asking our vendor some very pointed questions, we found out they had very few Spanish-speaking nurses and also that our members had to go through several steps on the phone with English speakers before they could get to the Spanish-speaking nurse."

TeleSalud, therefore, was developed in-house to insure control over the quality of the service. The health plan recruited widely for nurses, establishing both clinical and cultural hiring criteria as well as a salary scale attractive to experienced nurses. The current TeleSalud nurses are all registered nurses with backgrounds in critical care and emergency nursing. Most are in their forties or older and have at least twenty years of nursing experience, according to Kathy Williams, clinical manager of the advice line.

The extensive training that Temple interpreters receive to differentiate word usage by nationality occurs more casually at Molina, mostly at staff meetings or over lunch. TeleSalud nurses are predominantly Latinas, but their heritage is as diverse as that of Molina's members: Mexico, Guatemala, Peru, and El Salvador. Because the nurses work side by side in a call center, they're able to help each other out and share knowledge, for example, of medicinal teas that certain patients might use or about practices such as swaddling feverish infants.

"Our approach is one of support to the member, but we're doing medical triage at the same time, so it's important to inquire about any home remedies the patient is already employing," Williams says. "There's a wide range of calls. You have people who should have called 911 twenty minutes ago and you have people who just have a cold. With the second group, our aim is to discourage them from going to an ER and exposing themselves to more serious infection. But you have to use your clinical judgment. If that judgment is that the patient may come to harm, then the advice changes to 'I think it might be a good idea for you to go to the emergency room now.'"

TeleSalud was piloted in Southern California's San Bernardino and Riverside Counties, where many Latino members live, including new immigrants who have little experience with preventive care and tend to use emergency rooms in crisis. As TeleSalud began to get repeat callers, nurses took the opportunity to discuss things like immunizations and well-baby checkups, as well as follow-up care. The system has expanded since Hablamos Juntos to include a bilingual appointment-scheduling line to which nurses can transfer a caller if they judge that a physician visit is needed.

Other new services include after-hours prescription refills, case management for members with chronic conditions, and calls to patients who have been treated in ERs to make sure they follow up with their doctors. While each service is intended to help patients, each is also designed to reduce costs by preventing unnecessary ER use or exacerbation of illness, leading to expensive hospitalization. Molina calculates savings based upon analysis of the number of callers triaged by TeleSalud to alternate sources of care, whether it's a next-day doctor's appointment, a visit to an urgent care center, a consultation with a specialist in chronic disease management, or simply reassuring instruction on home care measures.

—⁓— Aftermath

Hablamos Juntos spurred the Robert Wood Johnson Foundation to once again reevaluate its approach to racial and ethnic disparities in health care. Program leaders realized that it wasn't practical or sufficient to "ask some poor hospital to just offer translation services" or to expect the federal government to pay extra for cultural competence, according to Anne Weiss, senior program officer and leader of the Foundation's quality/equality health care team. Instead, the Foundation's strategy has become one of folding the special needs of ethnic and minority patients into overall efforts to improve health care quality, whether that means giving medicine to patients who can't afford their prescriptions, arranging home nurse visits, or using an interpreter to help, say, a Chinese-speaking diabetic understand the dietary regimen.

In 2005, the Foundation authorized $3 million to support certain Hablamos Juntos activities through mid-2009. The same year, it launched a new program, Speaking Together: National Language Services Network, that was, in the words of Foundation assistant vice president Dickson, "more consistent with our philosophy of looking at better communications between non-English speakers and providers as one way of improving quality of care." Under the Speaking Together program, ten hospitals nationwide are working to identify, test, and assess strategies for effective language services in the context of overall medical care quality. Among early findings is the need for greater use of interpreters at key moments of information exchange—for example, at assessment and discharge—not just during the acute phase of treatment.[19]

Hablamos Juntos helped define this broader mission of language services as a contributor to health care quality through insights about communication deficits that extended beyond the program's targeted Spanish-speaking population. For example, in translating consent documents for surgery and other treatments, grantees discovered that the English versions were clotted with legalistic jargon that obscured important information about risks and benefits.

Other successor programs that opted for a more comprehensive approach include Expecting Success: Excellence in Cardiac Care, an $11 million program that ran between 2005 and 2009. Instead of trying to improve health outcomes via a limited focus on language assistance, as in Hablamos Juntos, Expecting Success worked from evidence that African American and Latino cardiac patients fared poorly due to a wide array of factors, including communication deficits, and it tailored remedies accordingly.[20]

Through Expecting Success, the Foundation also encouraged data collection on patients' ethnicity, race, language, and cultural characteristics in order to build an information base capable of pinpointing disparities and informing evidence-based solutions. "It's not enough to know that 80 percent of patients are getting good care across the board," Dickson says. "You want to know, is that 90 percent of white patients but only 40 percent of African

Americans?" She adds, "You have to think strategically about where this fits in a hospital's or other organization's gestalt, their operational game plan."

—∿— Conclusion

The last twenty years has seen considerable effort by government, philanthropy, and the private sector to improve cultural competence in the American health care system. Although knowledge of the influence of culture on health and health care has been around a lot longer than that, the activity of recent years has been prodded by a wave of new immigrants and mounting evidence of disparities in the health of people outside the American mainstream.

A landmark 1985 study by the Department of Health and Human Services documented persistent deficits in black and minority health.[21] This led in 1988 to the creation of an assistant directorship within the Centers for Disease Control (now called the Centers for Disease Control and Prevention) dedicated to minority health. The unit became the Office of Minority Health in 2002, and, three years later, the Office of Minority Health & Health Disparities (OMHD).

This evolution of OMHD parallels developments in the research field. What was once viewed as primarily racially based inequality in health care access and quality now is seen as multifactorial. The proof is OMHD's expanded mission, which today includes not only populations defined by race and ethnicity but also groups whose poor health correlates with socioeconomic status, geography, gender, age, disability, and particular risks related to sex and gender.[22]

Experiments like Hablamos Juntos have contributed to this broader view of population characteristics contributing to disparities in health and health care. The answers are complicated, intertwined, and not always amenable to precise measurement. As the Institute of Medicine found in its 2002 study, *Unequal*

Treatment, it's difficult to isolate a single factor—race, poverty, illiteracy, isolation, cultural beliefs—that if squarely addressed can be convincingly shown to improve the health of a population group.

Hablamos Juntos sought to tease out one factor—language barriers—for remedy with a variety of measures that health care organizations might be persuaded to invest in, especially if they resulted in cost savings from things like improved efficiency, reduced risk of complications from misunderstanding, and more appropriate use of health care services by patients with limited English proficiency. However logical this seemed at the outset, measuring impact proved difficult, partly because of the short duration of the Hablamos Juntos experiment—only two years to implement language improvements and conduct follow-up with patients—and partly because of the great variability of approaches tested by Hablamos Juntos grantees. Also complicating the analysis were significant differences in the characteristics of the Latino population each site set out to help. The two projects highlighted in this chapter—Temple University Health System's interpreter program and Molina Healthcare's Tele-Salud Advice clinical service—amply illustrate the difficulties of cross-site comparisons in assessing health impact and bang for the buck.

Perhaps because it was evaluated after only two years, Hablamos Juntos did not make the case for the cost-effectiveness of interpretation. Most private health insurers and government payers do not reimburse providers for these expenses. Tellingly, states with the largest immigrant populations and the most to gain from service improvement to patients with limited English proficiency have not taken advantage of federal options to reimburse the cost of interpreters through their Medicaid and CHIP programs. Absent solid evidence of savings elsewhere—Molina Healthcare stands out as an exception—cost remains a pressing concern for health care providers faced with growing numbers of uninsured patients and strained budgets. The situation is not likely to change soon, given the battered state of the American economy.

Results from Hablamos Juntos also raise questions about whether professional interpreters are the best option for non-English-speaking patients. Surveys of Latinos served by the project found that the majority preferred providers who spoke their language and, lacking that, some still opted for family members over interpreters. These are important findings that deserve further study.

Perhaps some of the health system's traditional ways of communicating with patients who have limited English skills deserve a second look. Old ways of doing things tend to get harshly judged in the excitement over a new approach. But is it really so bad for a bilingual physician to talk to patients in their native language, or for a bilingual nurse or clerk or family member to help out? Indeed, medical and nursing schools have invested heavily in promoting diversity in their student bodies to build capacity in the health care workforce to respond to patients' needs and preferences.

The needs of providers cannot be overlooked if the goal is to make language and cultural competence part of the standard of care in the United States. At Temple University Health System, erroneous assumptions about the medical staff's receptivity to interpreters led to several rough years for Temple's interpreters, and lingering tensions. Temple's Hablamos Juntos leaders, candid about their missteps in the spirit of helping others avoid them, say unequivocally that the medical staff should have been part of their planning process.

Hablamos Juntos demonstrated that effective communication is no less complicated and nuanced than many other factors underlying health and health care quality. Even people who are able to say exactly what they mean regardless of what pressures they are under can't be sure their messages are being received as they intend. Tone of voice, arms akimbo, wrong facial expression can send well-chosen words skidding into a bog of between-the-lines inference. Even when people speak the same language, emotion can sabotage comprehension. Patients have been shown to retain very little of the information that follows a serious diagnosis like "You have cancer." Personality traits lead some patients to exaggerate symptoms while others minimize them. Time pressures that define the modern health care encounter favor the terse over the long-winded, the distraught, the confused, and the silent. Still, patients with these idiosyncrasies—and many more—present daily in ERs, clinics, and doctors' offices.

None of this is to discount the importance of speech—or the contributions of Hablamos Juntos grantees in devising improved signage and educational literature in patients' native languages. There's no question that the health care system must address language barriers if it is to achieve overall quality goals. But context can't be overlooked. The Foundation's decision, post Hablamos Juntos, to incorporate language and cultural access into broader quality initiatives acknowledges this symbiosis and offers an opportunity to broaden the dialogue about communication in health care—a conversation enriched by the trials, errors, insights, and accomplishments of Hablamos Juntos grantees.

"We were a kind of Petri dish," says Yolanda Partida, Hablamos Juntos' national program director. "We were able to take a close look at language issues in a specific population of patients and, from that, learn a great deal about how to improve communication with all patients, not just those with limited English proficiency."

Notes

1. Institute of Medicine. *Unequal Treatment: Confronting Racial and Ethnic Disparities in Health Care.* Washington, D.C.: National Academies Press, 2002.
2. *Californians' Use of English and Other Languages: Census 2000 Summary.* Demographic Report Series no. 14, Center for Comparative Studies in Race and Ethnicity, Stanford University, June 2003. http://www.stanford .edu/dept/csre/reports/report_14.pdf. Accessed on June 12, 2009;

Hendricks, T. "43% in State Speak Other Than English at Home." *San Francisco Chronicle*, September 23, 2009.

3. "Improving Quality of Health Care Relies on Effective Language Services." An issue brief from *Speaking Together*. George Washington University School of Public Health and Health Services, October 2007. http://www.rwjf.org/files/research/speakingtogetherbrief102007.pdf. Accessed on June 12, 2009.

4. The Robert Wood Johnson Foundation. "Hablamos Juntos: Improving Patient-Provider Communication for Latinos" (call for proposals), 2001.

5. Morales, L. S., and others. *Language Access Services for Latinos with Limited English Proficiency: The National Evaluation of Hablamos Juntos*. Final report to the Robert Wood Johnson Foundation, RAND Corporation, March 20, 2007.

6. Chen, A. H., and others. "The Legal Framework for Language Access in Healthcare Settings: Title VI and Beyond." *Journal of General Internal Medicine, 22* (2 Suppl), 2007, S362–367.

7. *Federal Register*, Vol. 45, December 17, 1980, 82972 (notice).

8. *Federal Register*, Vol. 68, No. 153, August 8, 2003, 47311–47323.

9. Chen and others. "The Legal Framework for Language Access in Healthcare Settings."

10. Jellinek, P. S., and Isaacs, S. L. *Overcoming Language Barriers to Health Care*. Public policy case study. Los Angeles: The California Endowment, July 2007, p. 17.

11. Chen and others. "The Legal Framework for Language Access in Healthcare Settings," p. 365.

12. The foundation also funded Project Hope, to study economic and cultural barriers in access to care for Latinos; the University of Washington, to conduct a survey on cancer screening among Hispanic women; and the Emory University School of Medicine, to conduct an assessment of health literacy.

13. The Robert Wood Johnson Foundation. "Opening Doors: A Program to Reduce Sociocultural Barriers to Health Care." *Grant Results Report*, December 1998. http://www.rwjf.org/search/gsa/search.jsp?q=opening+doors&x=0&y=0&src=sw. Accessed on June 21, 2009.

14. The Robert Wood Johnson Foundation. "Hablamos Juntos" (call for proposals), 2001, p. 2.

15. Institute of Medicine, *Unequal Treatment*.

16. Morales and others. *Language Access Services for Latinos with Limited English Proficiency*.

17. Temple University Health System and Hablamos Juntos Program at Temple. *Confessions of a Linguistically Challenged Health System*. Philadelphia: Temple University Health System, September 30, 2005.

18. Quoted in the Robert Wood Johnson Foundation. "Temple University Health System in Philadelphia Improves Language Services for Spanish-Speaking Patients Through RWJF's Hablamos Juntos Program." *Grant Results Report*, October 2007. www.rwjf.org/reports/grr/048232.htm. Accessed on June 13, 2009.

19. "Improving Quality of Health Care Relies on Effective Language Services." An issue brief from *Speaking Together*. George Washington University School of Public Health and Health Services, October 2007. http://www.rwjf.org/files/research/speakingtogetherbrief102007.pdf. Accessed on June 12, 2009.

20. The Robert Wood Johnson Foundation. *Expecting Success Program Achievements* video. October 23, 2008. http://www.rwjf.org/quality equality/product.jsp?id=34774. Accessed on June 13, 2009.

21. Task Force on Black & Minority Health, US Department of Health and Human Services. *Report of the Secretary's Task Force on Black & Minority Health, Vol. 1: Executive Summary*. Washington, D.C.: US Government Printing Office, 1985.

22. Office of Minority Health & Health Disparities, Centers for Disease Control and Prevention. *About OMDHOMHD*. http://www.cdc.gov/omhd/about/about.htm. Accessed on June 13, 2009.

CHAPTER 10

MicheLee Puppets and the Fight Against Child Obesity

Digby Diehl

Editors' Introduction

Many programs funded by the Robert Wood Johnson Foundation aim at changing policy or developing innovative programs that have the potential to be picked up by government and expanded throughout the nation. Others have the more modest aspiration of simply trying to improve the health or health care of individuals. MicheLee Puppets, which is funded by the Foundation's Local Funding Partners program, is one of the latter—in particular, helping Florida school children lead healthier lives.

The Foundation long ago discovered that television, movies, and celebrities can be employed to deliver health messages. It is only a small step for puppets to do the same thing, following the lead of the Muppets, who have been educating young children since 1969.

As Digby Diehl, most recently the co-author with Bob Barker of *Priceless Memories* and a frequent contributor to the *Anthology* series, recounts in chapter 10, MicheLee Puppets travel throughout Florida, providing an entertaining—even rollicking—show for the state's schoolchildren. But the show is not just fun and entertainment. The puppets highlight ways that elementary school children can eat more nutritious food and be healthier. And the children bring that message home to their parents. MicheLee Puppets mesh nicely with the Foundation's priority of reducing the epidemic of childhood obesity in the nation.

If any readers are doubtful about the potential of puppet power, we urge them to watch the video of MicheLee troupe's Rico B. Kuhl's hip-hop rendition of *I Drinky Water*. It can be found on YouTube at *www.youtube.com/watch?v=vrXXcyyrTqE*. Once you've seen *I Drinky Water*, you'll think twice about drinking cola again.

It may seem preposterous to suggest that puppets can change the world, but puppets working for change pop into every nook, cranny, classroom, fireside, community hall, street, hospital room, refugee tent, doctor's office, and church around the world...A puppet's power is its inherent nature to "become" anything it's designed to be. Puppets synthesize ideas. They are the essence of a thought, concept, or character. They can teach without qualifications; model without ego, express without consequences. They can speak for us as a proxy.... When used with young audiences, they, being small themselves, can encourage children to face bigger things.

> Wendy Passmore-Godfrey
> Artistic Director
> W. P. Puppet Theater Society[1]

Since 1985, MicheLee Puppets in Orlando, Florida, has harnessed puppet power to bring educational theater to students in Florida schools. Its mission is "empowering lives through the art of puppetry," and over the last twenty-four years MicheLee Puppets has performed for more than 1.4 million children. With a repertoire that ranges from large, sophisticated stage productions to intimate performances for preschoolers, its offerings cover a wide range of challenging subject matter, including bullying, disability, divorce, nutrition, preserving the environment, global warming, literacy, and sexual assault.

The art of puppetry is as old as human history itself. Marionettes dating back to 2000 B.C. have been unearthed in both the Indus Valley and ancient Egypt, but other evidence suggests that puppetry may go back as far as 30,000 years—quite literally back to the Stone Age. European puppetry is rooted in the *commedia dell'arte* of the Italian Renaissance. Punch and Judy, *commedia*'s most famous British offshoot, dates back to the time of Samuel Pepys (1662), and eventually crossed the Atlantic to the New World. In the United States, the contemporary use of puppets for education blended with entertainment is embedded in the childhood memories of anyone old enough to remember *Howdy Doody*, *Kukla, Fran and Ollie*, Shari Lewis and Lamb Chop, or *Sesame Street*.

Since its inception, MicheLee Puppets has been using puppet theater to improve the lives of its audiences. The story of a little girl named Jacquee demonstrates the impact its performances can have. "We have a burn survivor puppet," says MicheLee Puppets' founder and executive director, Tracey Conner. "We do reentry programs for children who have been burned, when they go back to school. A few years ago, I got a call from the Burn Unit at the Orlando Regional Medical Center. There was a little girl named Jacquee who was going to a brand-new school, which is tough enough when you look like all the other kids, but Jacquee had been badly disfigured in a fire.

"They asked us to bring Lynne, our burn puppet, to the school. We were there on Jacquee's second day. We set up in the library, with about 150 third-graders seated on the floor. In front of them was just a table and a puppet, and we did our skit. The children got to ask Lynne questions about how she got burned, and how she felt about it. Just about every hand was up. They all wanted to talk to her and ask her questions about her situation. Finally, we pulled back and stepped aside, and Jacquee was introduced.

"She was this little tiny girl, and they placed a chair in front of all these kids. She bravely sat there and told her story. She explained that she and her brother and a cousin had been playing in a bonfire. One of the boys had picked up a stick and thrown it at her, and it caught her clothes on fire. 'I rolled on the ground, but I couldn't put the fire out in time,' she said. I remember a tear running down her cheek. You could have heard a pin drop on the carpet. The kids were just entranced with her.

"And then they got to ask her questions, which was magical. One of the kids wanted to know whether she was still mad at her brother and her cousin. Another wanted to know whether they came to see her in the hospital. These were sensitive, caring questions. After all that interchange was over, the kids all stood up and surrounded her and started hugging her.

"That was her second day of school. On her first day, nobody would talk to her. It wasn't because the children were mean. It was because they didn't understand. And the difference between Day 1 and Day 2 was a puppet.

"What we're doing is helping to create good little citizens," Conner says. "We're about teaching kids values at a young age, to inculcate those qualities so that when they grow up they are better human beings, and they are able to make healthy choices for themselves and to be respectful of other people."

Conner got into puppetry pretty much by accident. "I was in college in Ohio, at Bowling Green State University, studying acting and directing," she says. "I assumed that I would have a career onstage after I graduated. In my senior year, the local school district hired two of us theater students to go out and tour their schools with a set of Kids on the Block puppets." The Kids on the Block is a national organization that is still active today; it franchises out its puppets and its scripts to local groups all over the country. Most of its clients are service organizations, not puppetry professionals. These organizations put on plays that feature children with physical and mental disabilities—blindness, cerebral palsy, epilepsy, AIDS and HIV, among many others. Through puppetry, they help kids feel better about themselves and help other children become more accepting of them.

"When I came to Florida after I graduated," Conner continues, "I decided to do Kids on the Block here in Central Florida. I was twenty-two when I started the company, and had I known how hard it was going to be, I'm not sure I would have been brave enough to do it. It was something I knew how to do, but it was as much a financial decision as anything else. I called Michael Prazniak, who had been my puppeteer partner in Ohio. He was waiting tables—which is what you do when you're an actor in Ohio. He came to Florida and worked with me. The name MicheLee is a combination of our two middle names."

The Florida Diagnostic and Learning Resources System (FDLRS) was already using Kids on the Block to teach children with disabilities, but did so only sporadically and with regular teaching staff as puppeteers. Conner started training teachers for FDLRS to improve their puppet manipulation skills, then began making the rounds of the various elementary schools in the district herself, performing daily. In exchange, FDLRS promoted MicheLee Puppets in its newsletter. Conner then struck a deal with Florida Hospital in Orlando that allowed her to borrow its set of Kids on the Block puppets in trade for a commitment to visit the children's ward and perform once a month.

For Conner, it was a transformational experience. "You know, as a theater student I was all about the curtain call, and how much fun it was," she recalls. "But as a puppeteer, for the first time I realized that theater could be used to make a difference in someone's life. I saw how it touched the lives of kids and made a difference. It's what MicheLee Puppets can do. It's what I can do."

Prazniak worked with Conner for about a year, and then left to pursue other interests. "Michael had to earn a living, but I just kept going," Conner says. For her, "going" has meant a twenty-four-year history of developing and performing a series of highly acclaimed puppet plays for children of all ages. In 2003, MicheLee Puppets won the Marjorie Batchelder McPharlin Award, the puppetry equivalent of the Academy Award. For MicheLee, this puppet Oscar constitutes a nationwide honor from its peers, the Puppeteers of America, and was given in recognition of MicheLee Puppets' "outstanding contributions in the field of puppetry in education and therapy." Today, the troupe is a known and trusted brand name throughout the state of Florida. It was recently honored as the 2008 Walt Disney World Champions for Children by the Association of Fundraising Professionals of Central Florida.

Both the scope and the content of the plays are carefully geared to the age of the audience. When MicheLee goes to high schools, it offers *Every 90 Seconds*, which is not a puppet show but rather a tense drama with masks, dramatic lighting, and role-playing. Commissioned by the Victim Service Center of Orange County, the subject matter is very mature indeed, dealing with rape and sexual assault, and how victims can come forward and get the help they need.

"*Every 90 Seconds* often makes students uncomfortable," Conner admits. "But it's also making an impact. We're teaching teenagers about power and control and relationships, and that sexual assault is not about sex, it's about power. I direct the show. I helped write the show and I sit in the audience and cry almost every time I see it. You know there are real kids that are going through what the actors are portraying onstage."

The show has empowered any number of victims to come forward. "I remember one performance at a facility for children who have been removed from their homes due to abuse," Conner says. "Many of the girls in the audience were holding each other and crying throughout. Toward the end, one girl got up and left, and I worried that the performance had been just too intense for her. After the show, however, a case manager came over to talk to me. She told me that the girl had come over to her and said, 'O.K., I'm ready.' It was a significant step for her—she and her younger sister had been raped by their biological father over a long period of time, but she was having trouble with the idea of pressing charges against him. Seeing *Every 90 Seconds* gave her the courage to face her father in court."

The majority of MicheLee performances, however, are for elementary school children. Grades K through 5 may see *Rescuing Ruby Reef,* an underwater musical about a coral reef threatened by pollution. Youngest children (pre-K through second grade) may see *SomeBunny Special*, about self-acceptance and diversity, or *A Good Day for Pancake*, about bullying. There is also a show about bullying for older elementary school children (grades 3 through 5), but the approach is entirely different. Their program is called *BSI—Bully Scene Investigators*.

Without question, however, the star of the MicheLee repertoire is *EXTREME Health Challenge*, an off-the-wall whizbang audience participation game show about nutrition and fitness for grades K through 5. Although initially developed in 2003, it has been refined, revved up, and widely performed across Florida with the assistance and support of the Robert Wood Johnson Foundation.

—⌘— Childhood Obesity—A Burgeoning Problem

Since 1980, the United States has grown fatter at every level of society, across all age groups, geographic regions, and income levels. As of 2008, more than a fifth of all adults were obese in every state except Colorado. By comparison, in 1991, just seventeen years earlier, no state whatsoever had an obesity rate exceeding 20 percent.[2]

Unfortunately, children have been in the vanguard of this alarming trend. Over the past three decades, rates of childhood obesity have risen dramatically, more than doubling among very young children aged two to five and elementary school children aged six to eleven and more than tripling among adolescents between twelve and nineteen. Clearly, we are in the midst of a nationwide obesity epidemic.[3]

In a culture obsessed with thinness, many overweight children are mocked and taunted by their peers, and the emotional scars from this thoughtless cruelty can last well into adulthood. The health problems engendered by obesity, however, go far beyond depression and other personal self-esteem issues. Obese children are vulnerable to a host of what had formerly been considered adult health problems, including heart disease, high cholesterol, high blood pressure, and type 2 diabetes. "America's future depends on the health of our country," says Jeff Levi, executive director of the Trust for America's Health. "The obesity epidemic is lowering our productivity and dramatically increasing our health care costs. Our analysis shows that we're not treating the obesity epidemic with the urgency it deserves."[4]

Perhaps because of Florida's prominence as a retirement state, the obesity-related health issues of its children have not been allocated either the medical or the financial attention commensurate with their gravity. Although it ranks thirty-eighth out of fifty states in obesity rates among adults (23.3 percent), Florida has a considerably more serious childhood obesity problem, ranking twenty-first in the nation in obesity among children aged ten through seventeen (14.4 percent).[5] This statistic is even more significant because Florida ranks second only to Texas in the percentage of children who are not covered by health insurance (19.2 percent),[6] and fourth and third in the country in shortages of primary care and mental health care professionals, respectively. In other words, despite the fact that obesity is a significant children's health issue in Florida, neither the public nor the private sector appears to be devoting sufficient resources to begin tackling the problem.

Although poor nutritional choices have garnered most of the attention for their contribution to childhood obesity, lack of physical activity is equally to blame. Couch potato syndrome has hit Florida just as it has the rest of the nation. School-age children are especially vulnerable. As of 2005, more than 60 percent of Florida's high school students and more than 31 percent of the state's middle school students did not participate in any physical education at school. That same year, just under half (49.5 percent) of all middle school students watched television for three or more hours a day, and a fifth (20.5 percent) used the computer for fun for three or more hours. An additional 17.1 percent reported playing video games for three or more hours.[7]

School is the natural point of intervention to deal with both the nutritional and the inactivity components of the problem. "To halt the epidemic of childhood obesity, we don't need a tipping point," said Risa Lavizzo-Mourey, president and CEO of the Robert Wood Johnson Foundation. "We need a pivot point, and school is it. School is where our children spend their days and where they learn habits that stay with them for life."[8]

Schools, however, have been slow to improve the nutritional value of the meals they serve, and the federal government has been less than helpful. Under federal guidelines, jelly beans and popsicles have been banned because they have "minimal nutritional value." Snickers and Dove bars are permitted, according to Margo Wootan, director of nutrition policy at the Center for Science in the Public Interest, because they supposedly contain some nutrients.[9]

The State School Foods Report Card, issued in 2007 by the Center for Science in the Public Interest, gave Florida a B-minus overall.[10] The 2008 spike in food and gas prices and the 2009 recession have left school districts even more challenged in their ability to provide healthy meals. Broward County Public Schools, the district which encompasses Fort Lauderdale, serves 44,000 breakfasts and 138,000 lunches daily. In 2008, its cost to provide milk to schoolchildren soared by nearly 42 percent over the prior year. Caught between unwavering nutritional requirements and a federal mandate requiring school food programs to be self-sufficient, the district was forced to consider raising lunch prices and cutting costs to make ends meet. Among other measures the district chose to take was the substitution of white bread for whole wheat.[11]

This is the situation facing schools throughout the state, and throughout the country. The Miami journalist Lee Klein explains, "Public school food deteriorated during the decades of budgetary cost-cutting that began with the USDA's redefining ketchup as a vegetable to help the Reagan administration pare $1.5 billion from the national lunch program. The federal government purchases more than $800 million worth of farm surplus products each year and turns them over to the school lunch program. The USDA, which administers the system, considers this a win-win situation: Schools receive free ingredients, while farmers are guaranteed a steady income. Trouble is, most of the commodities provided have been bottom-of-the-barrel meat and dairy products laden with saturated fat and cholesterol. On the plus side, any kids who later in life end up in a penitentiary will probably find the cuisine behind bars comforting; the USDA sends prisons the same foods it delivers to schools."[12]

—⚌— A Connection Is Made

Although combating childhood obesity through a puppet show may seem like an unusual approach, it clearly had the potential to accomplish important objectives that were not being addressed at the governmental level. The connection between MicheLee Puppets and the Robert Wood Johnson Foundation was made through a conference in Orlando on curbing youth violence. "Ann Manley from the Dr. P. Phillips Foundation was hosting and organizing part of this meeting, and a reception was planned at the Victim Service Center," Conner recalls. "She invited MicheLee Puppets to perform part of our youth violence show *Choices* at the reception.[13] Patty DeYoung from the Darden Restaurants Foundation was also at the meeting, and introduced me to Jane Lowe from the Robert Wood Johnson Foundation. When I told Jane about our healthy lifestyles show, she invited me to submit a proposal through the Foundation's Local Initiative Funding Partners program. That proposal led to a $50,000 planning grant in 2004–2005.

—⚌— An Unconventional Grantee

One purpose of the planning grant was to hone and fine-tune the presentation of the existing healthy lifestyles show, which originally had been entitled *Extreme Game Show*. MicheLee Puppets consulted with nutritionists, pediatricians, and other specialists to sharpen the curriculum content. After its makeover, the show was renamed *EXTREME Health Challenge*. The initial planning grant also provided for the development of classroom teacher lesson plans focused specifically on nutrition and exercise. These guides are now pegged to specific sections of Florida's Sunshine State

Standards in subjects ranging from science and math to language arts, and give teachers a strong means of reinforcing the educational message of the puppet show. Matches for the planning grant were provided by the Edyth Bush Charitable Foundation, the Chatlos Foundation, Florida Hospital, SunTrust Banks, the Winter Park Health Foundation, the Community Foundation of Central Florida, the Darden Restaurants Foundation, and the Martin Anderson-Gracia Andersen Foundation.

Perhaps even more important, the planning grant also allowed MicheLee Puppets to take stock of itself from top to bottom, examining goals, structure, process, and resources. It enabled MicheLee to step up to become a more professional organization, and to institute methods and procedures by which it could support and sustain growth over the long term. A business/strategic plan, marketing and communications plans, and a long-range fundraising plan were all completed under the planning grant.

It was a giant leap forward for a small band of puppeteers. The total staff of MicheLee Puppets is just fourteen, including puppeteers, technicians, and office personnel. Only seven of the fourteen are full time. Everyone on staff multitasks. Denise Lucich started as a puppeteer and is now the communications manager. "I'm also IT tech, coordinator for the move into our new building, and fashion design and coordination," she says with a laugh.

"When we first met Tracey Conner, MicheLee Puppets was at a critical juncture," says Pauline Seitz, who was at the time the director of the Robert Wood Johnson Foundation's Local Initiative Funding Partners program (and is now director of a successor program called the Local Funding Partnerships program). "MicheLee Puppets was a small community organization that was well-respected and functioning well. When we made our initial site visit, we were impressed by Tracey's work, but at that point in 2004, the weight of a Robert Wood Johnson Foundation grant would have been far too much for her organization to bear. There was a lot of strategic planning work that they had to do to be ready, in terms both of developing their board and of business planning. She had to make some very deliberate decisions about what she wanted the future to look like. Since that time they have used every bit of support and advice that comes with a large organization like Robert Wood Johnson, and they have stayed closely connected to their local funders."

The philanthropic environment in Central Florida has greatly facilitated this connection. "Central Florida has for a long time been a place where people want to give back," says Ann Manley of the Dr. Phillips Foundation. "All of the organized philanthropies know about each other and know what the others like to do and not do, and we work together. With MicheLee Puppets, we have funded specific programs, specific scripts. We always get wonderful feedback from Tracey about how many performances they gave and how many children attended. She stays in touch."

Under the grant, MicheLee Puppets reached out far beyond its traditional base in Central Florida, partnering with other organizations across the state that are active in fighting childhood obesity. Once the revisions for *EXTREME Health Challenge* had been completed, MicheLee Puppets worked with its statewide partners to roll out the new and improved program in twenty-six schools. *EXTREME Health Challenge* premiered as a pilot program in the spring of 2005; responses and comments from teachers and audiences who previewed the show helped further refine it thereafter.

—〰— Florida Kids Take the *EXTREME Health Challenge*

After completing the planning process, MicheLee Puppets received a $360,000 four-year (July 2005–June 2009) implementation grant from the Robert Wood Johnson Foundation, through the Local Initiative Funding Partners program. The local funders that supported the planning grant also provided funds for the implementation grant, and MicheLee Puppets was able to bring a wide range of other funders on board.

Matches from the initial partners were supplemented by grants from the Aetna Foundation, the Florida Department of Health, the Mattel Children's Foundation, the Health Foundation of South Florida, and the Blue Foundation for a Healthy Florida, among others.

Grant monies were used to present *EXTREME Health Challenge* at elementary schools across the state. With the participation of Florida's ten regional Area Health Education Centers (AHECs), the neediest schools and school districts were prioritized for *EXTREME Health Challenge* performances. School participation in Florida's free and reduced-cost lunch program was used as a leading indicator. Although the intensity of the 2005 hurricane season forced the cancellation of a number of performances, by the beginning of the 2008–2009 school year, nearly 200,000 students at 413 schools in 35 of Florida's 67 counties had seen *EXTREME Health Challenge*.

What makes *EXTREME Health Challenge* so appealing and so memorable? The show makes a conscious effort to mimic the high energy, the frenetic pace, and the decibel level of video games and TV game shows—the very entertainments that keep children anchored and sedentary in their seats in the first place (and thus contribute to the problem). Although humor is ever present, the health message is equally clear.

Part *Who Wants to Be a Millionaire*, part *Jeopardy!*, and part *Fear Factor*, *EXTREME Health Challenge* directly involves members of the student body and offers them the chance to interact with a sextet of fuzzy, madcap puppets, including Zak the pogo-maniac, Kirk the ex-video game addict, and Babe the reformed sugar junkie. These puppet characters are all noteworthy in their own way, but the one who usually makes the biggest impression is the debonair ladies' dude and outlandish puppet-about-town Rico B. Kuhl. Rico is the bling-laden self-proclaimed—and self-absorbed—King of Reggaetón. "Calm down, ladies, calm down," he says as he makes his entrance. "There is plenty of Rico to go 'round." He then presents one of the hosts of the show with an unsolicited autographed head shot, "because I am so bee-yoo-teeful . . . Let's get on with this so my fans can adore me."

With his handsome lavender movie star visage, his suave Latin lover accent, and his perfectly coiffed shiny black hair, the ever-so-hip Rico is a walking advertisement for the health benefits of hydration. In addition to featuring him in *EXTREME Health Challenge*, MicheLee Puppets has also made him the star of his own music video called *I Drinky Water*. After he arrives on the scene in a cherry red classic convertible, an adoring chorus of girl groupies asks Rico "How did you get so cute?" He delivers his response in a Latino hip-hop rap style whose cadence is contagious:

> *My eyes so bright*
> *My hair so shiny*
> *My skin so soft*
> *Just like a baby's hiney.*
> *I take a little swig*
> *Everywhere I go*
> *They don't-a give me soda*
> *'Cause all the girlies know*
> *I drinky water*
> *I drinky water*
> *I drinky water*
> *Drinky drinky drinky drinky water. . .*

Along with posters and other promotional materials, *I Drinky Water* is distributed to schools to ramp up student enthusiasm for upcoming *EXTREME Health Challenge* performances. In addition to being aired regularly by the Florida Department of Education on the Florida Knowledge Network, the video also plays on YouTube.[14] Another promo music video features a tub-thumping, knee-slapping, Nashville-tinged ditty whose anti-preservatives message is trumpeted in its title: *If You Can't Read It, Don't Eat It*.

The need to drink enough water is just one topic covered in the half-hour *EXTREME Health Challenge* show. Others include the value of getting enough daily exercise—and the many different kinds of activities kids can choose from, how to make smart choices in packing a school lunch, the importance of eating lots of fresh fruits and vegetables rather than packaged foods, and how to read the nutrition label on a cereal box and what to look for: more whole grains, fiber, and vitamins, less sugar.

Even during *EXTREME Health Challenge*, however, there are opportunities to reinforce the self-esteem of children with mental and physical disabilities. At one school, a child named Blake was chosen from the audience to compete in the "Super Label Challenge" portion of *EXTREME Health Challenge*. In this segment, two students race on one foot to pluck phrases such as "Total Fat" or "Vitamins" from a giant nutrition label. Blake was one of those chosen, but he was different from his classmates. Blake had cerebral palsy; his movements were jerky and unsure. He could not run, or even walk very fast, and as a result, at recess no one would pick him for their teams—at least not until they saw him hopping on one foot in the challenge. His successful participation helped others in his class see him in a new light.

Part of the impact of MicheLee Puppets is that its performances are indeed theater. "We are artists," Conner declares. "We provide exceptional quality theater, especially for elementary school kids who don't always have the opportunity to see theater. We deal with many different topics, but at the core is the issue of respect for self and for others, and the need to take personal responsibility and make positive choices in your own life."

—⟋⟍— Measuring Results

EXTREME Health Challenge is undeniably entertaining, but how can anyone be sure that the message is getting through? The development of evaluation tools that would deliver a set of specific measurable outcomes was a key component of the planning grant. MicheLee Puppets hired professional consultants to design and test its evaluation technique. The result was two separate pre- and post-tests, one for kindergarten through second grade, and another for grades 3 through 5. These tests confirmed that children understood the message of *EXTREME Health Challenge*. After the first year of the program, children who had seen the show were able to answer at least 85 percent of the post-performance test questions correctly. During the second year, a revision to the post-test was added to measure intent to change and improve behavior with regard to diet and exercise. In the aftermath, test results indicated that at least 88 percent of children were motivated to improve.

MicheLee Puppets also videotaped several of its performances, recording not the actors and puppets onstage but the students in the audience. Carefully viewing the videos, staffers counted the number of times students looked away from the action for five seconds or more. Each diversion of five seconds was considered a loss of attention. They found that attention levels ranged from 98 to 100 percent. Simply put, the kids were glued to the stage.

"We started working with MicheLee Puppets years ago," says Patty DeYoung, foundation administrator for the Darden Restaurants Foundation, the nominating partner for the initial Robert Wood Johnson Foundation grant. "It's not until you go out and watch the awe on the children's faces and watch the magic that happens that you really understand the impact of what they're doing." "MicheLee Puppets is reaching kids with a very important message about health and physical fitness," adds Susan Black of Florida Hospital, one of MicheLee Puppets's funding partners. "They give children the knowledge and power to take control of their own health. That's what we love about the show."

These observations were verified by an evaluation of the first year's activities conducted by Valerie George, Research Associate Professor in Dietetics and Nutrition, College of Health and Urban Affairs, Florida International University. Several of the conclusions of the assessment are especially noteworthy. "In the book *The Tipping Point*, Malcolm Gladwell defines the 'stickiness factor' as the specific quality that a message needs to be successful and memorable," writes George. "Producers of *Sesame Street* built their program on the insight that if you can hold the attention of the children, you can educate them. A research team headed by Ed Palmer was able to measure the attention level of the program by individual segments. Scenes featuring the puppet characters had the stickiness factor, and were most effective in holding children's attention. The average attention for most shows was 85 to 90 percent."

—w— Hitting Home

Although measurement and testing have confirmed that the students are paying attention during the show and that they can answer the questions correctly in the immediate aftermath of seeing the program, some challenge whether this knowledge translates into real and lasting behavior modification. Teachers themselves are skeptical of the long-term benefits of the program, as indicated by their comments. "I don't think one day will change eating habits. Parents have a lot to do with it," and "The show helps, but is not the only thing that affects their choices."[15]

It does not help that at a time when schools are particularly hard-pressed financially they have turned to unusual sources of revenue to cover their costs. School vending machines filled with soft drinks and unhealthy snacks have historically been a revenue stream for schools. In the past, the Orlando area school district has sent home report cards in envelopes promoting McDonald's and offering a free Happy Meal to any student with a good report card. The practice is not unique to Orlando; other Florida districts have included coupons for pizza, free ice cream, and other fast-food items. Although schools choose to interpret these promotions as business partnerships rather than advertising, that distinction may be lost on families at home. Worse, it would appear to strengthen an unfortunate connection between good grades and the reward of fast food in the minds of young children.

In this environment, what effect can one puppet show have? After children have seen *EXTREME Health Challenge*, what changes take place in how they eat or exercise once they return home? After all, even with an avowed intention to make healthy dietary choices, children are not in control of their own nutrition. And, of course, once elementary school kids get home from school, they are up against a powerful interlocking conspiracy of bad influences, some deliberate, some accidental, some merely uninformed.

Commercial television programs still insistently market unhealthy food items, including sugary cereals and heavily processed salty snacks, to young viewers. Older teens share pizza and soft drinks with their younger siblings, giving them not only bad nutrition but also providing a poor role model in the process. A time-challenged working single parent may put fat- and preservative-laced foods, such as boxed macaroni and cheese, on the table in an effort to serve dinner—any dinner—quickly. There are monitoring and supervision issues as well. Whether in an after-school program or at home, an elementary school child watching television or sitting at a computer demands far less of an adult's attention than a child outside at play. Even for grade school children who have grasped the message of *EXTREME Health Challenge* and want to exercise and eat healthily, these pressures and influences may be difficult to overcome.

Despite all this, Conner is betting on puppet power. She is confident that the kids in her audiences are carrying the message home. "We took a package to the post office, and the mail clerk saw the MicheLee Puppets return address on the label," she recalls. "'Oh my gosh!' the clerk exclaimed. 'My kids saw your show, and they have been bugging me and my husband to go for a walk after dinner.'" In a sense, children who have seen *EXTREME Health Challenge* become little lobbyists for the new message of exercise and healthy eating. "Kids know what's good," Conner says, "and they will speak up to their parents." "Part of the answer has to be to involve parents," says Kathy Harper, senior manager, public affairs at Blue Cross and Blue Shield of Florida. "We're focused on the children, but Tracey is having an effect by reaching parents through them."

"An important part of the show is letting kids know that they have the power to make some choices by themselves," Conner insists. "They can choose to play outside rather than watch TV. They can choose an apple over potato chips. They can choose water over soda. I know because I've seen it happen; so have many members of my team." "Children leave the show cognizant that they have a choice," says the host and puppeteer Alex Lewis, who voices Rico, Zak, and Kirk. "That's our big thing—that kids have the power to decide what they're going to eat."

Every member of the troupe has heartwarming and even tear-inducing stories of individual children and their reaction to the shows. Following a performance, the actors were loading the *EXTREME Health Challenge* sets and equipment into the van when they were approached by a parent with tears in her eyes. "I just wanted to thank you," she said. "Yesterday, my little boy was getting off the bus when the driver told him, 'Hurry up, Fatty!' You see, my son Chris is obese. Devastated by the words of the bus driver, he refused to eat breakfast the next morning. That afternoon, he saw *EXTREME Health Challenge*, and learned that he had the power to make good health choices. He was so happy. 'Mom! I can eat less junk food. I can drink water instead of soda. And I can exercise every day!'"

"Chris went from feeling depressed and defeated to feeling excited and empowered to make healthy changes in his life," Conner explains. "That's the power of puppetry."

—∿— Lessons Learned: Building Sustainability through Prudent Management

It is a fact of life for MicheLee that those children who could most benefit from puppet power are those who can least afford to pay. Under the Robert Wood Johnson Foundation grant, schools were offered *EXTREME Health Challenge* at no cost. Looking ahead to the time when the Foundation is no longer underwriting the cost of presenting the program in Florida schools, MicheLee Puppets instituted a $300 fee for its shows. Even at that price, however, *EXTREME Health Challenge* is a bargain. For MicheLee, the average cost per school to put on the show is approximately $2,400.

"For the first couple of years, we had a shotgun approach with *EXTREME Health Challenge*, and we just went everywhere with the show," Conner says. "In these last months of the grant, we are focusing on areas where we can sustain the performances through other funding. We have a large potential in South Florida, and another in the Jacksonville area, where we have a partnership with the Jacksonville Children's Commission for their after-school program. With our major national grants like the Aetna Foundation and substantial statewide grants such as the Blue Foundation, we can hit other geographic areas as well. We may not do as many counties, but we'll still do as many schools."

The ability to prudently manage the growth and survival of the puppet company is an enduring legacy of the Robert Wood Johnson Foundation grant, in particular the 2004–2005 planning grant. Initially, however, that grant was something of a disappointment. "I confess that when we first found out about it, it was a bit of a jolt," Conner says. "My initial feeling was that they were giving us money to plan to do something we were already doing all the time. I didn't understand what more we needed to do."

Some of MicheLee's local funding partners were disappointed as well. "We were all set to go on the big grant when we got this letter," says David Odahowski, president of the Edyth Bush Charitable Foundation, a major supporter of the puppet company. "At first, it was a bit of a letdown, like a consolation prize. But in the long run it was terrific. This became Tracey's graduate course, her Ph.D. in nonprofit management, and it came from Robert Wood Johnson through the accountability that was built into the grant."

"The Robert Wood Johnson Foundation has caused us to raise the bar at every level," agrees the MicheLee communications manager, Denise Lucich. "It has caused us to think about every facet of what we do. We have made great improvements in how we present ourselves to the public—our press releases, our e-mails, our printed materials. And the training has been incredible. I've been through two different courses of communications training, and it causes you to open up to different perspectives, things you've never thought about. My head explodes whenever I go for training."

"I learned that I didn't know what I didn't know!" Conner exclaims. "Every time we've gone for seminars, it's opened up doors we might have been afraid to walk through—or doors we didn't even know were there. We are not the same organization that we were before we got the grant. I am not the same director or the same administrator that I was before the grant. We learned the importance of marketing and communications, and now have a line item in our budget for it. As a result of working with consultants, we learned how beneficial it is to bring in outside experts to help us do the things we can't do ourselves. We also expanded our network of funders and partner organizations, and we learned that it is O.K. to ask your funding partners for help other than dollars."

"On the operations side, we have learned how to protect our artistic integrity while demonstrating effective business practices," Conner says. "We have become diligent about becoming a self-sustaining organization. We know how to apply successfully for grants, we know how to approach the business community for support, and we have been successful in proving to the community just how valuable we are."

MicheLee Puppets has carefully built an expanding web of partnerships and alliances that will sustain them after their Robert Wood Johnson Foundation grant ends. "These other foundations, including Aetna and the Blue Foundation, came on as matching grants to the Robert Wood Johnson Foundation grant," Conner explains. "We have now established relationships with these foundations that are totally independent of Robert Wood Johnson, and those relationships are going to continue."

"I always tell grantees that Robert Wood Johnson is just a phase they're going through," Pauline Seitz says. "MicheLee Puppets' ability to forge these new relationships makes them an excellent example of how grantees should prepare to function independently after their grant period ends."

—∿— Looking Ahead: Replicability

Somewhat notorious among her supporters and funding partners for being financially conservative, Conner admits that the nation's economic downturn has slowed the implementation of some of the more ambitious growth and expansion plans for MicheLee Puppets. Right now, the primary focus is on staying fiscally sound, and on strengthening partnerships with foundations, public interest organizations, and other support groups. There are plans to broaden the reach of *EXTREME Health Challenge* and other MicheLee Puppets programs both within the state of Florida and into other states as well.

Because a funding partner has been secured, however, there will soon be an additional cast performing *EXTREME Health Challenge*. Partnering with Holy Cross Hospital in Fort Lauderdale, MicheLee Puppets will add another team of puppeteers based in South Florida. "This will save us thousands of dollars in hotel and per diem travel expenses," Conner says. "We will also be performing for family groups—kids and parents together. That will be something of an experiment, to see if it makes a difference in what happens at home after the children see the show. If it does, we may start doing that in other areas as well."

Another growth option is to find other groups of puppeteers who will buy the rights and do the show in their area. "We've been exploring this possibility with a puppet group in Georgia, but we are still in the talking stage," Conner says. "If we can do that and it goes well, we could license the show in other states as well." Conner does have concerns about losing creative control over the show once it is out of her hands. "I worry about making sure that whoever is performing *EXTREME Health Challenge* does a good job—about making sure that they will have the same positive impact on children that I know we have.

"We see our puppets as building bridges, opening doors," Conner says. "If you remember Jacquee the burn survivor, her story didn't end with her second day of class in third grade. Two years later, we were once again at her school performing. She was in the school office picking up homework, because she was on her way to the hospital for yet another surgery. Someone told her that MicheLee Puppets was in the library. She went to the library and hugged the puppeteers. She knew that we had made a difference for her."

Meanwhile, a new generation of parents, teachers, and health professionals is interacting with MicheLee Puppets at its performances—grown-ups who had seen the puppets as children. "Makes you feel old, and it makes you feel great at the same time," Conner says. "We were doing a show for foster children and one of the case managers came up after the performance. 'Tracey, I'm Jennifer.' It took a minute or two, but suddenly I knew exactly who she was. We had received a letter from this little girl. 'Dear MicheLee, I am handicapped. I can't see well. Sometimes I wonder why God made me this way. Then I think I am special, too. I give great hugs. And I have a friend who really cares about me. And then I think I'm glad to be me. Sincerely, Jennifer.'

"Jennifer had been a chubby little girl with glasses who had a learning disability. We had done a promotional videotape of her reading her letter. 'You know,' she said, 'your show was a turning point for me. I realized that I was smart, and that I could do things. And it changed the way I thought about myself.'"

Jennifer had gone on to college and become a social worker, helping other kids with problems. "These kinds of encounters are reason enough for me to keep doing this," Conner says. "I love my job every day, but I especially love my job on the days when a teacher, parent, student, past student, or community member approaches me to let me know that the service we offer is really making a difference."

—⁓— Little Miracles

"The success of *EXTREME Health Challenge* can help sum up what MicheLee Puppets has become, how we have grown as an organization, and where we would like to go," Conner says. "This show is another example of our direct-to-student approach for teaching important concepts through the power of puppetry. We really do get through to the kids."

The puppets sometimes can reach children when nothing else has worked. "Several years ago, I was the puppeteer doing *SomeBunny Special*," Denise Lucich recalls. "And I did a show for a group that included autistic children. Many of them had more than one handicap, and the sounds they were able to make were mostly grunts and groans. After the show ended, I invited the special needs teachers and students to stay, and I did a one-on-one with the children. When I brought out the bunny, the kids were grunting and groaning. Then I brought out the raccoon—more of the same. The aides had reassured me that these were really happy sounds. I brought out Howling Hound Dog, played with him, and then had him sniff the feet of the kids, and say, 'Woof. Woof.'" There was this one little boy—when I stopped at his feet and did the woof-woof thing, he turned around and said, 'Woof. Woof.'"

"To me it was no big deal, but then I noticed the teachers were all crying; the aides were hysterical. Someone said, 'Oh, I wish his mother was here!' It was the first word he'd spoken in four years. The puppets had gotten through to him. I know I could go other places and make a lot more money, but we get to see all these little miracles. I love what I do, and I love the message that we give, and I know we make a difference."

Notes

1. Passmore-Godfrey, W. *Puppet Power*. W. P. Puppet Theatre, 2007. www.wppuppet.com/pp2007_article_jan.html. Accessed on June 13, 2009; Passmore-Godfrey, W. "Message Audience Medium," address to plenary session, Puppet Power 2007—Puppets as Agents of Social Change conference, May 16–17, 2007. www.wppuppet.com/pp2007 _plenary.pdf. Accessed on June 13, 2009.
2. Trust for America's Health. "Florida Adults 34th Most Obese in Country; Youth 21st Most Overweight," press release for fourth annual F as in Fat: How Obesity Policies Are Failing in America conference, August 5, 2008. http://www.getoutdoorsflorida.com/Documents/Obesity%20Report%20 in%20Florida%202007.pdf. Accessed on June 13, 2009.
3. Trust for America's Health. *F as in Fat: How Obesity Policies Are Failing in America*, August 2008. http://healthyamericans.org/reports/obesity2008 /Obesity2008Report.pdf. Accessed on June 13, 2009.
4. Ibid.
5. Trust for America's Health. State Data: Florida, Key Health Facts. http://healthyamericans.org/states/?stateid=FL. Accessed on June 13, 2009.
6. Ibid.
7. Obesity Prevention Program, Florida Department of Health. 2005 Florida Youth Risk Behavior Survey (YRBS), Florida Department of Health Obesity Prevention Program, Current Trends and Statistics. http:// www.doh.state.fl.us/Disease_ctrl/epi/Chronic_Disease/YRBS/Topic_Fact _Sheets/Fact_Sheet_5_Weight_Management.pdf.
8. Alliance for a Healthier Generation. "Clinton Foundation, American Heart Association, Robert Wood Johnson Foundation to Help Schools Create a Healthier Environment for Nation's Students," press release, February 13, 2006. http://www.healthiergeneration.org/uploadedFiles /For_Media/afhg_nr_healthy_schools_2-13-06.pdf. Accessed on June 13, 2009.
9. Martin, A. "The School Cafeteria, on a Diet." *New York Times*, September 5, 2007. http://www.nytimes.com/2007/09/05/business/05junkfood. html?scp=1&sq=&st=nyt. Accessed on June 13, 2009.
10. Center for Science in the Public Interest. *State School Foods Report Card 2007*, November 2007. www.cspinet.org/2007schoolreport.pdf. Accessed on June 13, 2009.
11. Bushouse, K. "Soaring Food Costs Forcing Changes in Your Child's School Menu." *South Florida Sun-Sentinel*, May 7, 2008. http://www .sun-sentinel.com/news/local/broward/sfl-flbschoolfood0507sbmay07,0, 4342978.story. Accessed on June 13, 2009.

12. Klein, L. "Fast-Food Children: Making School Lunches Healthy Is an Uphill Battle." *Miami New Times*, January 10, 2007. http://www .miaminewtimes.com/2007-01-11/restaurants/fast-food-children/. Accessed on June 13, 2009.

13. *Choices* was a youth gang violence show for middle school audiences that is no longer in the MicheLee Puppets performance rotation. It was suspended after the school shootings at Columbine in Colorado. "We just stopped. What was edgy all of a sudden was not edgy enough," says Conner. "It was nothing compared to what kids were really dealing with. We haven't gotten back to this issue, but we will."

14. MicheLee Puppets. *Rico B. Kuhl—I Drinky Water, EXTREME Health Challenge* video, 2007. http://www.youtube.com/watch?v=vrXXcyyrTqE. Accessed on June 13, 2009.

15. Valerie George, *Final Evaluation Report of Year One (of MicheLee Puppets)*, 2007–2008.

—⟋⟍—The Editors

Stephen L. Isaacs, JD, is a partner in Isaacs/Jellinek, a San Francisco-based consulting firm, and president of Health Policy Associates, Inc. A former professor of public health at Columbia University and founding director of its Development Law and Policy Program, he has written extensively for professional and popular audiences. His book, *The Consumer's Legal Guide to Today's Health Care,* was reviewed as "the single best guide to the health care system in print today." His articles have been widely syndicated and have appeared in law reviews and health policy journals. He also provides technical assistance internationally on health law, civil society, and social policy. A graduate of Brown University and Columbia Law School, Isaacs served as vice president of International Planned Parenthood's Western Hemisphere Region, practiced health law, and spent four years in Thailand as a program officer for the US Agency for International Development.

David C. Colby, PhD, is the vice president of research and evaluation at the Robert Wood Johnson Foundation. Previously, he was the deputy director of research and evaluation, the deputy director of the health care group, interim team leader for the quality team, and team leader for the coverage team at the Foundation. He came to the Foundation in January 1998 after nine years of service with the Medicare Payment Advisory Commission and the Physician Payment Review Commission, where he was deputy director. Earlier he taught at the University of Maryland Baltimore County, Williams College, and State University College at Buffalo. Colby's published research has focused on Medicaid and Medicare, media coverage of AIDS, and various topics in political science. He was an associate editor of the *Journal of Health Politics, Policy and Law* from 1995 to 2002. He received his doctorate in political science from the University of Illinois, a master of arts from Ohio University, and a bachelor of arts from Ohio Wesleyan University.

—∿—The Contributors

James Bornemeier is a writer with more than twenty-five years experience in journalism as an editor and correspondent at the *Providence Journal, Philadelphia Inquirer,* and *Los Angeles Times,* where he shared in a staff Pulitzer Prize. He is now a New York City-based writing and editing consultant, working primarily with major philanthropic organizations such as the Ford Foundation, the Robert Wood Johnson Foundation, and the Goldman Sachs Foundation. From 1997 to 2003, he worked at The Pew Charitable Trusts where he oversaw communications for the culture and public policy programs. He is a graduate of Northwestern University.

Michael H. Brown was a reporter for the *Louisville Courier-Journal* for twenty-eight years, the last seventeen as Washington correspondent. Since leaving the newspaper in 1997, he has been a freelance writer, focusing largely on health care but also occasionally on the less weighty realm of outdoor recreation, including boating, biking and hiking. He is a graduate of Wesleyan University and received a master's in journalism from Northwestern University. He and his wife, Margaret, have five grown children and live in Arlington, Virginia.

Digby Diehl is a writer, literary collaborator, and television, print, and Internet journalist. His book credits include *Priceless Memories,* the bestselling autobiography of Bob Barker; *Remembering Grace,* a look back at the life of Grace Kelly (with Kay Diehl);

the recent novel *Soapsuds,* written with Finola Hughes; *Angel on My Shoulder,* the autobiography of singer Natalie Cole; *The Million Dollar Mermaid,* the autobiography of MGM star Esther Williams; *Tales from the Crypt,* the history of the popular comic book, movie, and television series; and *A Spy for All Seasons,* the autobiography of former CIA officer Duane Clarridge. For eleven years, Diehl was the literary correspondent for ABC-TV's *Good Morning America,* and he was recently the book editor for the *Home Page* show on MSNBC. Previously the entertainment editor for KCBS television in Los Angeles, he was a writer for the Emmys and for the soap opera *Santa Barbara,* book editor of the *Los Angeles Herald-Examiner,* editor-in-chief of art book publisher Harry N. Abrams, and the founding book editor of the *Los Angeles Times Book Review.* Diehl holds an MA in theatre from UCLA and a BA in American studies from Rutgers University, where he was a Henry Rutgers Scholar.

Lee Green is an independent writer and journalist. Based in Ventura, California, he has pursued stories in Europe, Canada, Central America, the Caribbean, and throughout the United States. The results of those labors have appeared in a diverse array of magazines, from the *Atlantic Monthly* and *Audubon* to *Sports Illustrated, Los Angeles, Playboy,* and *Outside,* where as a contributing editor and columnist he wrote frequently on health, fitness, and human performance. One of his pieces, a story about Death Valley, published by American Way, won the Lowell Thomas Award for the year's best article on US travel. Several of his articles have appeared as cover stories for the *Los Angeles Times Magazine.* Notable among these are a critique of the US Forest Service; a look at America's secular ethics movement; an open letter to Governor Arnold Schwarzenegger citing the inequities of California's famed Proposition 13 property tax law; and an illumination of California's failure to prepare for the state's projected population growth. Among his current projects is a book on US foreign policy.

Robert G. Hughes, PhD is a vice president of the Robert Wood Johnson Foundation and its chief learning officer. Since joining the Foundation in 1989 as director of program research and then vice president, Hughes has played an instrumental role in program development and management in tobacco control, children's health insurance, tracking health systems change, and community health projects. Hughes is currently responsible for the Pioneer Portfolio, the component of the Foundation dedicated to promoting fundamental breakthroughs in health and health care through innovative projects, including those from nontraditional sources and fields. Before joining the Foundation, Hughes was an assistant dean at Johns Hopkins University. He also taught at the University of Washington School of Public Health and Community Medicine and the Arizona State University College of Business. Hughes received a PhD in behavioral sciences from Johns Hopkins University and a Pew postdoctoral fellowship in health policy at the University of California, San Francisco. He received an MA from Ohio State University, and a BA from DePauw University.

Risa Lavizzo-Mourey, MD, MBA, is the fourth president and chief executive officer of the Robert Wood Johnson Foundation, a position she assumed in January 2003. Under her leadership, the Foundation implemented a defining framework that focuses its mission to improve the health and health care of all Americans and set bold objectives in nursing, health care disparities, and childhood obesity as well as improving public health and quality in the health care system. She originally joined the Foundation's staff in April 2001 as the senior vice president and director of the health care group. Prior to coming to the Foundation, Lavizzo-Mourey was the Sylvan Eisman Professor of Medicine and Health Care Systems at the University of Pennsylvania, as well as director of the Institute on Aging. Lavizzo-Mourey was the deputy administrator of the Agency for Health Care Policy and Research, now known as the Agency for Health Care Research and Quality. Lavizzo-Mourey is the author of numerous articles and several books, the recipient of many awards and honorary doctorates and frequently appears on national radio and television. A member of the Institute of Medicine of the National Academy of Sciences, she earned her medical degree at Harvard Medical School followed by a master's in business administration at the University of Pennsylvania's Wharton School. After completing a residency in internal medicine at Brigham and Women's Hospital in Boston, Massachusetts, Lavizzo-Mourey was a Robert Wood Johnson Clinical Scholar at the University of Pennsylvania, where she also received her geriatrics training.

Fred Mann, assistant vice president of communications for the Robert Wood Johnson Foundation, works closely with David Morse in managing the Foundation's strategic communications efforts. A longtime print and online journalist and manager, Fred coordinates the activities of Foundation communications officers and staff, oversees Web operations, co-chairs the Foundation's Editorial Policy Board, and serves on the Program Executive Group which is responsible for the oversight of all grant making and program strategies. Before coming to the Foundation, Mann spent twenty-three years with the *Philadelphia Inquirer* as features editor, Sunday Magazine editor, and assistant managing editor. He also created and ran the newspaper's Web site, Philly.com, one of the first newspaper online operations, and he served the newspaper's parent company, Knight Ridder, as vice president for national programming for the chain's twenty-eight Web sites. Prior to working in Philadelphia, he was national editor of the *Hartford Courant* and a reporter for *The Day* newspaper of New London, Conn. He also created a syndicated west coast news service that provided coverage to a dozen major papers including the *Boston Globe, Newsday,* the *Miami Herald,* and the *Detroit Free Press.* He has reported for *Time Magazine* and other national journals, and served as a press secretary in the US Senate for three years. He is a graduate of Stanford University with a BA in communication.

David Morse has been vice president for communications at the Robert Wood Johnson Foundation since 2001. In that role, he has created a new approach to communciation, emphasizing speaking with and on behalf of grantees to maximize awareness and impact of Foundation goals and programs to promote Foundation policy objectives. From 1997 to 2001, he was director of public affairs for The Pew Charitable Trusts, responsible for managing the Trusts' relationships with media and policymakers and with advising grantees on communications strategies. Before joining Pew, Morse served as associate vice president for policy planning at the University of Pennsylvania, building the university's relations with the federal government, leading efforts to create new mechanisms for financing higher education, promoting tax policies that preserve incentives for charitable giving, and teaching public policy at Penn's Graduate School of Education. As an aide to US Senators Jacob Javits and Robert Stafford, Morse developed legislation affecting higher education and cultural affairs for the Senate Committee on Labor and Human Resources, and in 1981 directed the President's Task Force on the Arts and the Humanities. He received a BA from Hamilton College and an MA from The Johns Hopkins University. He serves on the Ad Council's Public Policy Advisory Committee.

Tony Proscio is a freelance writer and a consultant to foundations and nonprofit organizations. His recent clients include the United Nations Secretariat, the Ford, Rockefeller, Surdna, and McKnight Foundations, the Atlantic Philanthropies, the Nonprofit Finance Fund, and the Local Initiatives Support Corporation. He is coauthor, with Paul S. Grogan, of the book *Comeback Cities: A Blueprint for Urban Neighborhood Revival,* published in 2000 by Westview Press, which Ron Brownstein described in the

Los Angeles Times as "the most important book about cities in a generation." He is also the author of *In Other Words, Bad Words For Good,* and *When Words Fail,* three essays on civic and philanthropic jargon published by the Edna McConnell Clark Foundation. In separate *New York Times* columns, William Safire described *In Other Words* as "a gem," and Jack Rosenthal cited its "skillful verbal archeology." From 1995 to 1997, as New York City's Deputy Commissioner of Homeless Services, Proscio had chief operating responsibility for New York's forty emergency shelters caring for 35,000 homeless adults a year. In Miami, he established Homes for South Florida, a bank consortium for community-development lending, and later became associate editor of the *Miami Herald,* where he was lead editorial writer on economic issues and wrote a weekly opinion column.

Sara Solovitch is a writer whose stories have appeared in *Esquire, Wired, Outside,* and other publications. She has been a staff reporter at several major newspapers, including the *Philadelphia Inquirer,* and has had numerous stories published in the *Washington Post* and the *Los Angeles Times.* For six years, she wrote a weekly column on kids' health for the *San Jose Mercury News.* She has taught writing and journalism at all levels—from elementary school to the graduate program in science communication at the University of California Santa Cruz. Currently, she's an editor at *Bay Area Parent,* and her magazine stories have won national awards from the American Society of Journalists and Authors, the National Education Association, and Genetic Alliance. She lives in Santa Cruz, California.

Irene M. Wielawski is an independent writer and editor specializing in health care and policy topics. She has written extensively on socioeconomic issues in American medicine, particularly the difficulties faced by people without timely access to medical services because of financial, geographic, cultural, and other barriers. Wielawski was a staff writer for nearly twenty years for daily newspapers, including the *Providence Journal-Bulletin* and the *Los Angeles Times,* where she was a member of the investigations team. Subsequently, with grant support from the Robert Wood Johnson Foundation, she tracked local efforts to care for the medically uninsured following the demise of President Clinton's health reform plan. Other commissioned projects include producing segments for public television on pediatric medicine topics and an analysis of the Massachusetts health reform law. Her independent work has been published in the *New York Times* and the *Los Angeles Times,* among daily newspapers, on Web sites, and in peer-reviewed journals and books. Wielawski has been a finalist for the Pulitzer Prize for medical reporting, among other solo honors, and shared in two *Los Angeles Times* staff Pulitzers. She is a founder and current board member of the Association of Health Care Journalists, a reviewer for *Health Affairs,* an outside editor for the *American Journal of Nursing,* and a graduate of Vassar College.

—ᴡ—Index

—◠◠—Anthology Chapters by Topic 1997 through Volume XIII

Health Insurance Coverage, Access, and Cost

Overview Chapters

The Politics of Health Care Reform, Vol. XII (2009)

Research on Health Insurance Coverage, Vol. XII (2009)

Efforts to Cover the Uninsured, Vol. IX (2006)

Safety-Net Programs, Vol. IX (2006)

Cost Containment, Vol. VII (2004)

Health Services Research, Vol. XI (2006)

Managed Care, 2001

Workers' Compensation, 2001

Academic Medical Centers, 1998–1999

Medical Malpractice, 1997

Data Collection/Analysis

National Access-to-Care Surveys, 1997

Health Tracking, Vol. VI (2003)

State and Local Levels/Increasing Enrollment

Enrolling Eligible People in Medicaid and SCHIP, Vol. XII (2009)

Improving State Government Capacity in Health Reform, 1997

Medicaid Managed Care, Vol. IX (2006)

The Covering Kids Communication Campaign, Vol. VI (2003)

Health Insurance for Children, 2000

Health Insurance and Small Business: The Communities in Charge
Program, Vol. IX (2007)

Rural Areas

Improving Health Care in Rural America, Vol. XII (2009)

Primary Care in Rural Areas: The Practice Sights Program, Vol. VI (2003)

Encouraging Physician Volunteerism: The Reach Out Program, 1997

The Southern Rural Access Program, Vol. IX (2007)

The Swing Bed Program, Vol. VI (2003)

Access to Specific Services

Tuberculosis Care, Vol. V (2002)

Dental Care, 2001

Community-based Dental Education: the Pipeline, Profession and Practice Program, Vol. XII (2009)

Mental Health: The Chronic Mental Illness program, 2000

Mental Health Services for Youth, 1998–1999

Emergency Medical Services, 2000

AIDS, Vol. V (2002)

Asthma, Vol. XII (2009)

Health Policy/Public Policy

The National Health Policy Forum, Vol. VII (2004)

Shaping Public Policy as a Foundation Approach, Vol. XII (2009)

End-of-Life

SUPPORT, 1997

The Foundation's End-of-Life Programs, Vol. VI (2003)

Public Health

The Turning Point Program, Vol. VIII (2005)

Responding to Emergencies: 9/11, Bioterrorism, and Natural Disasters, Vol. VII (2004)

Substance Abuse/Addiction Prevention and Treatment

Tobacco

The Foundation's Tobacco-Control Strategy and Initiatives, Vol. VIII (2005)

Tobacco Policy Research, 1998–1999

The National Spit Tobacco Program, 1998–1999

The Sundance Conference and its Aftermath, 2000

Tobacco Cessation, Vol. VI (2003)

Smoking Cessation and Pregnant Women (The Smoke-Free Families Program), Vol. XI (2008)

The National Center for Tobacco-Free Kids, Vol. VI (2003)

The SmokeLess States Program, Vol. VIII (2005),

Drugs and Alcohol

The Foundation's Efforts to Combat Drug Addiction, Vol. XIII (2010)

The College Alcohol Study, Vol. XIII (2010)

The Evolution of the Foundation's Efforts to Prevent and Treat Addictions, Vol. IX (2006)

Community Anti-Substance Abuse Coalitions (The Fighting Back Program), Vol. VII (2004)

Supporting Anti-Substance Abuse Coalitions (CADCA and Join Together), Vol. VII (2004)

Working with Head Start (The Free to Grow to Grow Program), Vol. IX (2006)

Reducing Underage Drinking, Vol. VIII (2005)

Recovery High School (Albuquerque, New Mexico), Vol. V (2002)

Alcohol and Work: Results from a Corporate Drinking Study, 1998–1999

Obesity

The Active Living Programs, Vol. XI (2008)

MicheLee Puppets, Vol. XIII (2010)

Children and Adolescents

Quality/Equality of Care

Human Capital

Workforce Development

Fellowships and Scholarships

Nursing

Vulnerable Populations

Homeless People

The Homeless Families Program, 1997

The Health Care for the Homeless Program, Vol. IX (2006)

The Homeless Prenatal Program, Vol. VII (2004)

Minorities

Increasing Minorities in the Health Professions, Vol. VII (2004)

The Minority Medical Education Program, 2000

Overcoming Language Barriers to Care (Hablamos Juntos), Vol. XIII (2010)

Native Americans

Programs to Improve the Health of Native Americans, Vol. V (2002)

The Catholic Social Services Outreach Project in Lakota Sioux Reservations, Vol. XII (2009)

Fighting Back and Healthy Nations in Gallup, New Mexico, Vol. VI (2003)

People in the Criminal Justice System

Former Prisoners Reentering Society (Health Link), Vol. XII (2009)

Young People with Addictions in the Juvenile Justice System (Reclaiming Futures), Vol. XIII (2010)

Older People/Long-term Care

Programs on Aging, Vol. IX (2006)

Adult Day Centers, 2000

Faith in Action, 1998–1999

Long-Term Care Insurance Partnerships, Vol. IX (2007)

Consumer Choice in Long-Term Care, Vol. V (2002)

The Teaching Nursing Home Program, Vol. VII (2004)

Financing Affordable Long-Term Care Housing: The Coming Home Program, 2000

Integrating Acute and Long-Term Care for the Elderly: On Lok and PACE, 2001, 2001

Service Credit Banking, Vol. V (2002)

Measuring Unmet Need in the Community: The Springfield Study, 1997

Demystifying Philanthropy

Learning from Foundation-funded Programs

Learning from Programs that Did Not Meet Expectations, Vol. XIII (2010)

Redesigning Programs in Mid-Course, Vol. XIII (2010)

The National Health Care Purchasing Institute, A Case Study, Vol. XIII (2010)

The Role of Failure in Philanthropic Learning, Vol. XIII (2010)

Inside the Robert Wood Johnson Foundation

The Foundation's Early Years, Vol. VII (2004)

The Foundation: 1974–2002, Vol. IX (2007)

A Ten-Year Retrospective: 1997–2006, Vol. IX (2007)

An Interview with Steven Schroeder, Vol. VI (2003)

Expanding the Focus: Health as an Equal Partner to Health Care, 2001

Adopting the Substance Abuse Goal, 1999

Program-Related Investments, Vol. V (2002)

Grantmaking in New Jersey, Vol. V (2002)

Research as a Foundation Strategy, 2000

National Programs as an Approach to Grantmaking, Vol. VIII (2005)

Engaging Coalitions as a Foundation Strategy, Vol. IX (2007)

Communications

Communications Strategy at the Robert Wood Johnson Foundation, Vol. XIII (2010)

Getting the Word Out: A Foundation Memoir and Personal Journey by Frank Karel, 2001